Psiloc

Mushr

A Step by Step Guide to Growing, Microdosing and Using Magic Mushrooms

Ronald O'Neil

Disclaimer Notice:

Please note the information contained within this document is for educational and entertainment purposes only. All effort has been executed to present accurate, up to date, and reliable, complete information. No warranties of any kind are declared or implied.

Readers acknowledge that the author is not engaging in the endearing of legal, financial, medical, or professional advice. The content within this book has been derived from various sources.

Please consult a licensed professional before attempting any techniques outlined in this book.

Table of Contents

Introduction

There are rising numbers of people developing psilocybin mushrooms at home. Home cultivation eliminates the risk of misidentification of wild mushrooms in addition to a reliable supply throughout the year. It's also a fun, low-cost hobby for many growers.

You might be tempted to start with a psilocybin mushroom kit if you do not know how to grow mushrooms at home. These ready-to-use packages contain a living mycelium substrate (the material underlying the growth of the mushrooms) that you only have to keep moist in theory.

In fact, from scratch, you're better off. Making your own substrate is not only more coherent, but it should also be less contaminating if you do it correctly. There isn't a huge price difference, too, and you'll get to learn a lot more.

Psilocybin mushrooms are fungi containing the natural psychotic psilocybin compound, which is capable of producing intense hallucinations and spiritual encounters as well as other effects. More commonly referred to as "magical mushrooms" or "shrooms," psilocybin contains more than 180 species of mushrooms or its derivative psilocin. At the same time, fungi have a long history of spiritual and religious ritual use in Mesoamerica. These are also one of the most commonly used and popular psychedelics in the United States and Europe.

Nevertheless, psilocybin mushrooms are not only a drug and sacrament. They have been used in therapeutic environments to treat several ailments and disorders, including headache of clusters, obsessive-compulsive disorders, anxiety, depression, post-traumatic stress disorder, and dependence, and the recent resurgence in therapeutic effects of psilocybin showed promising results.

Chapter 1

Biology Of Mushrooms

Let us imagine this situation, a cow paw on a grassy field on a dairy farm somewhere in the sun-drenched tropics. A single, magnificent specimen of Psilocybe cubensis stands at the top of this cow patty. His stalk is robust and feathery straight, and his cap is open, flat as a dinner plate. For the whole world, the cow patty seems to have somehow got a parasol to shade itself against the devastating effects of the sun. A black, dark, and almost infinite cloud of spores rains out of the darkness to locations unknown with any turning wind. However, keep this picture at the back of your mind as you read this chapter, which contains many things you need to know about mushroom biology.

This chapter includes a lot of complicated details and scientific jargon. You can only think of wading knowledge on the nature and biology of fungi. Then again, perhaps you are delighted to explore new fields of scientific knowledge. However, we ask you to help us, as knowing the fundamental processes in the mushroom life cycle can explain the cultivational techniques we present. When and when something doesn't suit the plan, this knowledge will allow you to understand what you see so that you can change your approach accordingly.

This chapter is about the elimination of misunderstandings as well as the introduction of new knowledge. That is because most of us believe we understand the mushrooms and how they work in the

universe, and most of these ideas are false. When we first tried to grow mushrooms, we assumed we knew all about it, and our efforts were not quite spectacular. We only found success when we began to understand their mysteries.

What is a Mushroom?

Very few of us have anything to do with fungi, at least not with a choice. This is just like anything else, a cultural phenomenon. When most people believe in mushrooms, they picture the bland and harmless surfaces on their pizza or the exotic, ornate toads of a fairy tale and myth whose mere taste would drive a crazy person, if not kill him entirely. Mushrooms are fearful of poison or harmless vegetables for the vast majority of North Americans, and they do not deserve much thought. Even if you're in the tiny minority for which mushrooms provide fascination, wonder, and pleasure (probably due to one or more experiences with Psilocybe species), in your high school or college biology classes, you've probably learned little-by- little.

So, what is a mushroom exactly? A truffle is just one part of a fungus, not anything in itself, as you and your left elbow: w are related, but not the same. Strictly speaking, the reproductive structures of some mushrooms are roughly the same as the flowers of an apple tree, which contain "sowings" of future trees. Mushrooms are neither animal nor plant nor animal but are related to both. Not surprisingly, the correct classification of these elusive and hidden beings has always been subject to a lot of uncertainty. Most of us think of mushrooms and fungi as an odd variety of plants, often as they come from the ground like plants and seem incapable of

walking (or dancing or swimming) as lucky animals can do. It is the most significant misunderstanding most of us have about fungi and the one you need to dispense with immediately. Here it is also: fungi are not plants, and developing mushrooms are not like gardening. Fungi are not animals either, although they are closer to animals than plants, given their appearances. Plants, algae, and certain bacteria synthesize their energy, carbon dioxide, and water and are known as autotrophs. All other organisms, including fungi, are heterotrophic, which means that they are derived from plants or food products (say, fish) or food items that eat plants (larger fish). However, this is almost where the similarities between animals and fungi end.

Classification and Taxonomy of Fungal

To order to understand how fungi fit into the "animal, vegetable and mineral" order, the more formal systems biology you use is to classify Y species, which are known as Linnaean taxonomical (the first Swedish botanist and physician to establish Carolus Linnaeus). Every single species has a specific Latin double (or binomial) name like Psilocybe basis or Homo sapiens in this framework. Such two names apply to the last two categories-genus and species-of an eight-part hierarchy organized by

Divisions, to be larger than smaller, are country, kingdom, phylum, class, classes, families, genus, and species. The simplest way to understand this is by acting:

The most appropriate ranks to be addressed for our purposes here are a nation, genus, and species. Five kingdoms, and the fungi, the Kingdom Fungi, exist in themselves. Although there are many

variations on the topic, the one thing that all mushrooms have in common is that they digest out their food and absorb the component nutrients into their cells. All fungal species described in this book are in the Psilocybe genus.

Finally, each species has a special binomial, including Psilocybe cubensis or Psilocybe azurescens.

Types of Psilocybin Mushroom

The most well-known and eaten species are the 180 + known forms of psychedelic mushrooms:

• Psilocybin cubensis: The most famous and widely cultivated psilocybin mushroom.

• Psilocybe cyanescens: Slightly smaller and slightly more psychoactive than psilocybe cubensis, but not less cultivated.

• Psilocybe azurescens: This is probably the most potent psilocybin mushroom in the world, as discovered by world- renowned mycologist Paul Stamets in the mid-90s.

• Amanita Muscaria (Fly Agaric): A red and white mushroom that contains ibotenic and muscimol as psychoactive elements; this mushroom has been commonly used by the indigenous Siberian and Baltic cultures in shamanic practice.

The Life Cycle of a Fungi

It helps to understand what fungi are specifically for a living, how they get around, and what kind of love they lead living. One best way to do this is to trace the fungal cycle of life, the journey from birth to death, which is continuously repeated with each next generation. Understanding organisms' life cycles is an excellent way of sorting out what is unique to each of them as no two species act in the same way. Sexual reproduction is the recombination of two-parent individuals' genetic material into another. Each parent's container of genetic material is known as a gamete. The fungal gametes are called spores. A spore is a compact, protected cell that stays alive but sleeps for a long time until it finds a suitable home. All the fungi we discuss in this book are known as Basidiomycetes since they produce their spores on basidia, tiny baseball-bat-shaped protuberances lining their gills, blade-like structures arranged on a radial motive on the underside of the cap, or pileus.

Parts of the Mushroom

- Spore Discharge

Let's return to the lonely mushroom of our cow patty. Zoom closer: deep in the dark, millions of baseball-shaped microscopic basidia emerge from the flat sides of the gills lining the underside of the parasol, and four ovoid purple-black spores stand on the broad side of each basidium. Each spore is placed like a cap on a miniscule horn-shaped protuberance on the outside of the basidium, known as sterignta. Thanks to the evaporative cooling on the sun-struck head face of the cap, the air around the gills are moist and much cooler than around the mushroom. As the air cools, water condenses around the spore and its little stand, where a droplet starts to form.

The droplet grows until it supports its own structure, its surface tension breaks and the water from the droplet spread over the spore 's body. The power of this action attracts the spore to the sterigma. The sterigma, being somewhat elastic, collapses under the spore's weight only to move the spore back from its perch to the open space, beyond the face of the gills, by equal force opposite. The amount of force is calculated precisely to whistle the spore as far as possible, but not to the extent that it hits the face of the spore. It succumbs to gravity and is straight down and out under the bottom of the mushroom, where it is carried away with a little luck by a wind breeze, along with millions of its brothers and sisters. When the wind in our field subsides, two spores have settled down from our mushroom on a grass plot where they now wait patiently for an electron scanning microphone of psilocybe cubensis to get them back together for someone or somebody.

-     Fungal Growth

Now, imagine a cow, perhaps the one who pawned the cow at the beginning of the chapter. The cow is mumbling at our field because cows want to, and sooner or later, they are eating the blades of grass on which our single spores are lying, mingling them with lunch. Entirely swallowed by the grass, their digestive tract is swept only to emerge at the other end sometime later. Fortunately, the spores are resilient and well blinded and have no harmful effects on the cow's lid.

More than that, they feel smoking for their difficulties in the center of their favorite food piles: cow shit.9 Each of our spores germinates soon afterward; the cells are split and developing gradually into the tasty and nutrient-rich materials in the patty of the cow.

Growing fungi consist of hyphae networks: tubular filamentous cells spreading and dividing at their forward tips and often joining to build structures like forks or tan. Hyphae masses are known collectively as the fungal mycelium. Fungal mycelium frequently appears in the naked eye as white, fuzzy, or hair-like growth on the food source surface, as you can see on the underside of an elevated log. Most fungi spend their majority of days like an undifferentiated mycelium, creating specialized and complex structures like mushrooms occasionally.

Hyphal growth is also invasive, which means it occurs inside and often all over the substratum. Digestive enzymes separated into the environment from the tips of advanced mycelium degrade the substrate into simple organic molecules that the mycelium can absorb or engrave as it progresses. In reality, fungi digest out. While we eat our meals in the comfort of our own interior, fungi prefer to eat out.

The saprophytes or saprobes all of the fungi we discuss in this book indicate they derive their nutrition from non-vivid organic matter, in this case, dead or decaying plants. In comparison to parasitic fungi that colonize and eat living organisms and, in the final analysis, often destroy their host, mycorrhizal fungi live in symbiosis with their hosts.

Fungal Reproduction Part 1: Mating

Our spores, which have now developed into two of mycelia colonies, continue to explore the cow's pie, penetrate slowly, absorb its contents, and blindly reach each other. Eventually, their colonies will touch mycelium, and finally, our two lovers will meet. Yet their good fortune so far is no guarantee that they can tie the knot because fungi are just as picky as we humans when it comes to whom they choose as their partners. Fungi produce spores of various mattress styles to reduce inbreeding and to encourage genetic diversity. The matting styles are roughly equal to our two sexes, except that the number of fungi can vary from 2 to many thousands! "For our lovers (and our story) to mate, they are very compatible, and it's nothing less than love at a glance.

To this end, the cells of each of the individual mycelium are monocaryotic: their cells contain just one haploid nucleus, with only one-half of the genetic material of a mature fungus.

Our two fungi lovers are eventually merged into a single entity, a mature fungus, and now that our fungus is mature, it can do what mature mushrooms like feed. Fungi invade the substratum of the cow patty, with thick, ropy strands of mycelium, until the food supply has been drained from the food available, or any other environmental change causes it to create mushrooms.

Part 2:

Fruiting

All that remains now for us to return to a full circle is for our fungus to produce mushrooms with a new generation of spores. Just why and when mushrooms are formed is somewhat mysterious, and the reasons vary significantly between species. Some do so due to weather variations such as heavy rain, an increase or decrease in temperature, or both. Other fruits are produced only after the substrate is completely colonized, and nutrients are depleted. In all these cases, the fungus is probably caused to reproduce by the increasing probability of its own destruction. Still, other species wait years for fruit, only after subtle changes have occurred in the environment. Fortunately, Psilocybe cubet1sis is a promiscuous species and requires little encouragement for us. Under a variety of environmental conditions, the robust P. cubensis strains fruit easily and abundantly.

Many psilocytes, like Psilocybes, want to ensure their caps' vertical orientation to optimize spore release elevation and output.

Therefore, the fruit with the sunlight as a catalyst at the upper surfaces of the substrate. When the mycelium of our fungus has penetrated the top layers of the cow patty, tiny knots of hyphae develop at various points on the animal's exposed surface.

These hyphal knots soon develop into primordia (singular, primOJ;dium), also known as pins or pinhead, and eventually become miniaturizing, full versions of the whole mushrooms. It is during the pinning stage that the fungus sufficiently differentiates and develops several distinct types of cells. The top surfaces of the minuscule caps darken, while the cells that make up the shell, strip, gill, and veil separate and direct themselves appropriately within the primordial. Divide and collect the nuclei while surrounding walls (or septa) build a dense matrix of compacted cells. A mature primordium contains all the cells in the fully cultivated champagne; all it has to do is take up the water and expand it. If it does, it happens quickly and practically bursts.

In the rapid growth process, the natural properties of the mushroom begin to take shape. The stipe stretches out, the spherical cap is expanded, and the partial veil is then flattened, a small membrane that protects itself from the fragile gills. The cap extends when the gills are fully formed. The mask is then separated from the outside of the cap. Veil remains also hanging loosely like a small scarf, known together as an annulus, attached to the stem.

The lengthening mushrooms use light, air, and gravity to direct their caps as vertically as possible, ensuring an efficient release of the spores as soon as the gills expand. Millions of basidia grow on gills' vertical faces in a dense layer of cells known as hymenium. When the basidium matures, the haploid nuclei fuse into one diploid nucleus, and the sexual act that started when our two spores met is finally completed.

But this phase is short-lived, as this nucleus quickly splits and constructs four genetically unique, haploid daughter nuclei. These nuclei pass into the stergimata and are incorporated and deposited as spores at the end of the basidium. They wait for the moment to fly and fur our story to start once more.

Mushroom Cultivation Genetics

Hopefully, now, you can understand how most basidiomycete fungi are behavioral in a natural environment and how they are cultivated artificially. The situation has changed, but the biology remains the same. Many fruits, millions of spores per fruit, and perhaps hundreds or thousands of strains per generation, a certain small percentage of which will thrive, are the best results of the success of nature. On the other hand, at any point in the cycle, the cultivator succeeds by carefully choosing only the best candidates for further growth and by operating within a controlled (sterile) environment. The cultivation of mushrooms takes place in three main phases irrespective of mushroom species: germination or isolation, expansion, and finally fruiting. The first step is to isolate a mushroom culture from spores or tissues of a living mushroom. Spores germinated on nitrified agar in Petri dishes lead to a diversity of strains (after mating).

Within the same family, a genetically similar parent mushroom results in tissue culture. In any case, the growth of the fungal medium results in the dikaryotic mycelium. The cultivator can easily test for desired characteristics on the culture and detect contamination if present by using a semi-solid agar medium.

The mycelium can spread on agar indefinitely and can be stored at cold temperatures for later recovery at this point. After a sufficient clean crop has been extracted, the mycelium is transferred in quarter-sized stem jars into the secondary medium, typically sterilized whole grain. This stage is intended to expand the volume of mycelium in the final phase to an amount that supports the desired amount of fruit. In a wedge of agar, a small amount of mycelium is removed from the plate and deposited on the grain. The mycelium is extracted from the grain. Every few days, the grain jars are shaken to facilitate colonization.

When the grain is completely colonized, it is then employed to inoculate larger grain containers to further increase the mycelial mass, typically in sterilizable plastic bags. The material produced in this process is commonly known as spawning.

Once the appropriate medium is prepared (sterilization at this stage is generally not required, even if the substratum is pasteurized sometimes), it is mixed with spawn and left to colonize. After it is colonized, the fruiting substratum is begun. Once again conditions of initiation are specific to the species. Still, they generally include covering the substrate with a layer of non-nutritive, moisturizing material such as peat moose (called case layer) and mode) ringing the temperature, humidity, air exchange and light on the iridescent surface to create conditions for mushroom formation.

However, in case all goes according to plan, the mushrooms first appear as primordia, then they grow up in full size within a few days and begin to release their spores.

Chapter 2

What Is Psilocybin Mushroom?

Magic mushrooms - Psilocybin (4-phosphoryloxy-N, N-dimethyltryptamine) and psilocin are chemical compounds obtained from several forms of dried or fresh hallucinogenic mushrooms grown in Mexico, South America, and the southern and northwest regions of the United States. Psilocybin is classified as an indole-alkylamine (tryptamine). Such compounds have a similar structure to lysergic acid diethylamide (LSD) and are exploited for their hallucinogenic and euphoric effects to produce a "trip." Hallucinogenic (psychedelic) effects are possible because of the central nervous system (CNS) serotonin (5-HT) receptors.

Apparently, there are over 180-species of mushrooms that contain the chemicals psilocin and psilocybin. Just like the peyote (mescaline), hallucinogenic mushrooms have been used in native or religious rituals for decades. Both psilocin and psilocybin can also be manufactured synthetically in the laboratory.

However, there have been reports that psilocybin bought on the streets can actually be other species of mushrooms laced with LSD.

Brief History of Psilocybin Mushroom

Sahara Desert Archeological evidence shows that humans have been using psychedelic mushrooms for seven thousand years, and older and fungi are found in prehistoric art in many geographical areas. In most cases, they are known as religious symbols, mostly in ceremonies marking passage rights. Some people have thought the experience may have influenced prehistoric culture, from art to religion to social values that govern everyday life, if our ancestors used champagne.

Many people take this idea very far. In the '90s, Terence McKenna, an ethnobotanist and psychonaut, posed a "Stoned Ape Hypothesis," which suggests that early humans and pre-human hominids took psychedelic mushrooms and triggered intellectual advances that lead to evolutionary benefit — including the mind as we know it today. However, it should then be noted that due to a lack of evidence, the scientific community views this hypothesis with skepticism.

Throughout the Maya and Aztec culture of Mesoamerica, Mexico, and Guatemala, however, there are detailed records of pre- Columbian use of psilocybin. After conquering these regions in the 15th and 16th centuries, the Spanish banned indigenous people from using psychedelic mushrooms, finding them a wild and uncivilized cultural practice.

Notwithstanding this, indigenous shamans have secretly defied Spanish rule for over 400 years and have continued using and treating these mushrooms to protect their cultural heritage.

Psilocybe semilanceata, a psychedelic mushroom that their father had unwittingly collected and cooked in stews, was accidentally fed by four children in the west as the first reliable account of the "toxification" of psilocybin mushrooms.

First, isolated psilocybin isolated in a lab in 1957 by the famous Swiss chemist Albert Hofmann (who synthesized LSD) from

Psilocybe Mexicana, a mushroom species found primarily in Central America. A year later, it was first produced synthetically.

J.P. former vice president, Gordon Wasson. Morgan & Company was fascinated by psilocybin mushrooms and became obsessive. In 1955 he visited Oaxaca, Mexico, and met Mushroom shaman Maria Sabina, who introduced him to Psilocybin mushrooms.

Maria was a member of the indigenous Mazatec Indian tribe. During his first mushroom ride, he felt as if his soul was scooped out of his body.

In 1957, Time Magazine published his photo essay "Finding the Magic Mushroom," where he outlined his observations and effectively kickstarted the psychedelic mushroom movement in the west.

Timothy Leary and Richard Alpert, scientists at Harvard University, created a Harvard Psilocybin Project following the reading of Wasson 's experiences, then traveled to Oaxaca to taste psilocybin champagne. They did what visionary scholars in 1962 would have done without work: they started a psychedelic movement. Psilocybin mushrooms were rapidly taken into counterculture in the 1960s.

In 1971 psilocybin was classified as a Schedule I substance in the

U.S. by the United Nations Convention on Psychotropic Substances, making it illegal for all purposes.

However, the psilocybin mushrooms were not included in the United Nations Convention, which allows countries to sign the Treaty (essential of a Treaty) to control psilocybin-containing mushrooms as they find fit. In most countries, however, psilocybin mushrooms are illegal, although there are exceptions.

Psilocybin Therapy

The House will consider the fact that three psilocybin therapy trials are currently ongoing in the United States as proof of the favorable properties of psilocybin. These studies were supported by the Heffter Research Institute and the Psychedelic Studies Multidisciplinary Association. They were approved by the various office abbreviations (e.g., the FDA, DEA, etc.), which exercise strict control over the use of entheogenic substances in the U.S. Given the very draconian US drug legislation, such studies would be incomprehensible if psilocybin were genuinely dangerous. The studies investigate the potential use of psilocybin to alleviate the mental anguish of patients with end-stage cancer, treat obsessive-compulsive disorder, and treat cluster headache syndrome. What other therapeutic applications psilocybin has remains to be seen.

Future of Psilocybin Mushrooms

If the law is in place, it is unlikely that psilocybin mushrooms collect more than a small consumer base. After all, a fresh mold is physically different from commercially bottled alcohol and lacks the 'allure' of mass-produced illegal laboratory drugs, for example, cocaine or branded ecstasy pills. In other words, the intrinsic features of a fungus do not attract a mass audience. Pills, powders, and packaged medicines such as alcohol are, irrespective of legality, "customer-friendly," while a mushroom is a very emblem of "non-refinement." The mushroom can not 'dry one's sorrows.' Instead of decreasing self-awareness and self-awareness like alcohol, it raises awareness. The majority of the people seem to prefer a "quick fix," a "fast food," or simply to become blind drunk for reasons specific to our culture. The mushroom, however, by its very nature, does not

attract this very reckless side of the human psyche and thus has remained a fairly low-key pursuit over the last 30 years or so.

After all, it is prudent to examine the current trade-in mushrooms. The trade is currently fully self-governed. Instead, it would be better to regulate and license the trade. It would also be in the public interest to provide consumers with information of some kind. That, I guess, is a reasonable way forward, and I hope the House can look forward to this constructive opportunity. Export regulation and licensing suggest smart control, a strategy that is a complicated strategy to criticize any side of the political clasp.

Research of Psilocybin in England

MAPS collaborated with other researchers in the United Kingdom.

On the construction of the questionnaire to be completed at many points of purchase across the UK by purchasers of fresh mushrooms. The questionnaire will evaluate the positive and negative effects of fresh champagne. The final round of criticisms of the questionnaire was completed, and the data collection process will start in a matter of weeks. The study should take approximately four months to collect and analyze data.

We want to present the results of the study to the House of Lords / Commons in the hope that some direct data will be useful in the development of government policies.

Research of Psilocybin in the United States

MAPS is currently funding an ongoing FDA-approved study on psilocybin in the treatment of obsessive compulsion disorder (OCD) under the supervision of Dr. Francisco Moreno, University of Arizona,

Tucson, together with the Heffter Research Institute. Prompt results are promising. Also, MAPS actively support case reports and medical history of about 75 individuals with cluster headaches who used (illegally) and examined their clinical results on a web site (clusterbusters.com), and the case study that led to the Harvard Medical School, under the guidance of the Harvard Medical School.

Psilocybin Risk Analysis

While no drug is free, the profile of psilocybin is relatively small. There is no significant risk of physical damage to either body or brain by psilocybin. This is well established in over 40 years of research. MAPS has produced digital PDF versions of virtually all the groundbreaking research papers published on psilocybin to support this inference. Psilocybin 's neurological effects are usually well tolerated; they are milder than traditional psychedelics such as LSD, DMT, and ayahuasca; and are not related to hallucinations. In general, psilocybin users report pleasant recreational experiences and an improved understanding of themselves and the world. Users also witness spiritual/mystical experiences. The use of psilocybin leads to the mental health of the vast majority of users or is not at all beneficial. Psilocybin may cause mental instability in people who are prone to such problems. Even among mentally healthy individuals, psilocybin can present great psychological difficulties with continuous adverse effects until the subconscious material which has emerged in consciousness is addressed and integrated, in a way somewhat similar to dreams.

In contrast, such adverse effects can rarely occur in mentally healthy people. In approximately 1 in 5 million cases (a rough estimate), the issue of psilocybin reactions has resulted in suicide. While it is not clear that the beneficial effects of psilocybin are likely to prevent deaths than harmful consequences.

Current Usage of Psilocybin Mushrooms

•   Psilocybin mushrooms are the most widely used among younger and older people.

•   A study of 409 students in the northeast of the US in 2012 found that almost 30 percent of psilocybin mushrooms were at least once tested.

•   Reports from data collected in the 2010 National Drug Use and Health Survey (NSDUH) show that psychedelics — those including LSD, PCP, peyote, mescaline, psilocybin mushroom, and MDMA — were used by about 1.2 percent of people aged

12 and over in the last month, compared to other drugs. Ironically, the use of "psychotherapeutics" (such as prescription antidepressants and antipsychotics) is estimated to be nearly six times the rate of psychedelics illegally.

•   Surveys in 12 EU countries. Member States find that the use of psilocybin mushrooms for people between 15 and 24 years of age ranges from less than 1% to 8%.

•   In England, in 2004/2005, about 340,000 people aged 16-59 had been using psilocybin mushrooms just before being wholly illegalized in the UK.

Myths About Psilocybin Mushrooms

- Psilocybin Mushrooms Cause Brain Bleeding, Bleeding Of The Stomach, And Renal Failure

A stroke, hemorrhage, or aneurysm would be diagnosed as a "sanitation brain." There is no evidence that these mushrooms are ever causing stomach bleeding after the ingestion of psilocybin mushrooms. A 1981 report found that dilated pupils and excessively sensitive reflections were the two most common complications of mushroom use. Many literature reviews found no risks in healthy people linked to mushroom use.

As for kidney problems, the problem is an identifying problem for mushrooms. Psilocybe semilanceata does not cause kidney problems, but mushrooms in the family Cortinarius are frequently mistaken for P. semilanceata and damaged to the kidneys.

- Shrooms Make You Crazy

Researchers have identified similarities between mushroom psilocybin trips and psychotic episodes, such as those in schizophrenia, but this is temporary (the term "trip" in almost all cases). Those admitted into the emergency room after taking psilocybin mushrooms return within hours to their usual physical and mental states. Also, a large population study has found that classical psychedelics, such as psilocybin mushrooms and LSD, are not likely to suffer from emotional distress and suicide.

Although there is no conclusive evidence to suggest that psychedelic use may exacerbate potential mental health problems, many researchers believe this is the case. Therefore, you might want to avoid psychedelic drugs if you have a history of mental illness (especially schizophrenia).

-      Magic Mushrooms Are Toxic

If you categorize a chemical substance that induces a poisonous state and alters your awareness, and causes some change in your physiology as deadly, then surely, psilocybin mushrooms are toxic. But if this is the case, all drugs, including alcohol, tobacco, marijuana, and caffeine, are toxic. However, psilocybin would not be categorized as such in a narrower definition of a poisonous substance.

While non-psychedelic mushroom poisoning can lead to severe physical illness and, in rare cases, death, psilocybin mushrooms are not toxic. Therefore, it is critical to correctly classify mushroom types.

Frequently Asked Questions on Psilocybin Mushrooms

Question: Is it possible to detect psilocybin in the drug test?

Answer: The most common drug tests do not contain psilocybin mushrooms and metabolites. They are, however, rarely included in extended drug screens

Question: Could psilocybin cause emotional trauma?

Answer: If you follow the psychedelic 6S and stop psychedelic taking while your family is associated with mental health issues, psilocybin does not cause psychological distress.

Sometimes, psilocybin, if you don't follow 6S, can lead to a short period of acute psychosis, known colloquially as a "bad trip." While no concrete evidence exists, some scientists suspect that psilocybin may lead to potential mental health problems.

Question: How do I know if I have mushrooms with psilocybin?

Answer: Many mushroom species contain psilocybin, and some look like toxic mushrooms so that your mushrooms are appropriately identified. Many psilocybin champagne species can be recognized by their long, thin stalks and short conical caps.

Question: Is it legal to cultivate psilocybin?

Answer: Psilocybin mushrooms are illegal to possess, buy, or grow in most countries. However, in many places, spores can be purchased unless you use them to improve champignons.

Question: How do I consume psilocybin mushrooms?

Answer: Mushrooms of psilocybin can be eaten whole, brushed into tea, or cooked in milk. A mild dose of 1-2.5g can be measured on a single scale.

Question: How should I use psilocybin mushrooms to microdose?

Answer: Psilocybin mushrooms can be microdose with an intake of about 0.05-0.25 g, but the tolerance of all is different.

Question: How does the tolerance of psilocybin work?

Answer: A moderate dose of psilocybin is immediately tolerant. If you retake the medication soon, the result will be weaker. You should wait between psilocybin doses for at least three days.

Question: Can I use other medicines to mix psilocybin?

Answer: Psilocybin should not be mixed with Tramadol since it can lead to the syndrome of serotonin. Be careful when mixing cannabis, amphetamines, or cocaine with psilocybin.

How It Feels, Tastes, And Smells

What Does It Feel Like?

Most toxic mushrooms appear very similar to 'magic mushrooms,' and it is easy for pickers to confuse them. People have become seriously ill or have suffered by consuming a toxic mushroom.

Magic mushroom is often sold fresh or dry. In the UK, the most popular forms are liberty caps (Psilocybe semilanceata) and fly agaric (Amanita muscaria).

•   Liberty caps appear like tiny tan-colored mushrooms

•   Fly agarics appear like toadstools in red and white.

It's important to realize that certain forms of magic mushroom are better than others. For example, the fly agaric champagne is typically more effective than the mushroom cap.

One way to take magic mushrooms is liquid psilocybin. It is made of psilocybin, the psychedelic medicine that occurs naturally in mushrooms, which is a clear pale-brown color. It is available in bottles (small bottles).

How Does It Smell/Taste?

The caps are usually eaten raw and have a strong earthy taste and rubber-like texture – which makes them very chewy.

They don't taste as though they were frying mushrooms at home, so certain people seek to mask the flavor with an omelet or tea.

How do People Consume It?

-        By eating it

After picking, liberty caps are often eaten raw or are dried out and stored. People tend not to eat raw mushrooms because they can make you feel very sick.

-        By drinking

Some people make tea from dried mushrooms.

-        By Taking Liquid Psilocybin

Liquid psilocybin is produced by removing psilocybin, the naturally occurring endogenous compound present in mushrooms and liberty caps.

How Does It Feel Like?

How Do You Feel About It?

The intensity of magic mushrooms differs depending on their freshness, the season, and where they emerge. The power of magic mushrooms is rather difficult to estimate.

For most people, the world appears distorted when they take mushrooms. Also, time, colors, sounds, and artifacts may all look quite special.

Some people have slight visions, which are often called 'visuals.'

Taking magic mushroom will make you feel:

- Extremely giggling
- Euphoric
- In appreciation for individuals and stuff around you
- Energized
- Awakened

You will even hear it:

- Paranoid
- Anxious
- Panicked
- Overwhelmed

- Vomiting

What you feel will be influenced by how much you carry, your environment, who you're with, and how relaxed you are around them, as well as by your mood.

And if you're in a poor mood, feeling nervous or anxious, the magic mushrooms may only make those feelings worse.

How Does It Make People React/Behave?

This depends on the amount of magic mushrooms the individual takes. You may not even notice that a person takes a small dose of mushrooms.

People consuming greater doses of champagne will behave unpredictably. You can laugh a lot, pin yourself on other issues, be depressed or be suspicious.

Strategies for Psilocybin Use

Psilocybin mushrooms have long, thin stems that may seem white or grayish bested by tops with dim gills on the underside. Dried mushrooms are normally a rosy rust earthy colored shading with separated zones of grayish. Mushrooms are ingested orally and might be made into a tea or blended into different nourishments. The mushrooms might be utilized as new or dried items. Psilocybin has an unpleasant, unpalatable taste.

An "awful trip," or a disagreeable or, in any event, frightening experience, may happen with any portion of psilocybin. As a rule, dried mushrooms contain about 0.2% to 0.4% psilocybin and just follow measures of psilocin. The run of the mill portion of psilocybin utilized for recreational purposes fluctuates, with top impacts happening in 1 to 2 hours, and going on for around six hours.

Portion and impacts can fluctuate extensively, relying on the mushroom type, strategy for planning, and resilience of the person. It tends to be hard to decide the specific types of mushroom or how many psychedelic drugs each mushroom contains. Introductory littler portions and a more drawn out timeframe to decide the impacts might be a more secure alternative in case you decide to utilize psilocybin for recreational purposes.

Effects of Psilocybin Mushroom Use

Psilocybin impacts are like those of different stimulants, for example, mescaline from peyote or LSD. The mental response to psilocybin use incorporates visual and sound-related pipedreams and a failure to recognize a dream from the real world. Frenzy responses and psychosis additionally may happen, especially if enormous dosages of psilocybin are ingested.

Stimulants that meddle with the activity of the mind substance serotonin may modify:

- Mood

- Sensory perception

- Sleep

- Hunger

- Body temperature

- Sexual conduct

- Muscle control

Physical impacts of psychedelic mushrooms may incorporate a sentiment of queasiness, spewing, muscle shortcoming, disarray,

and an absence of coordination. Joined use with different substances, for example, liquor and cannabis can uplift, or exacerbate these impacts.

Different impacts of hallucinogenic medications can include:

- Intensified feelings and sensory encounters

- Changes in a feeling of time (for instance, time passing by gradually)

- Increased circulatory strain, breathing rate, or internal heat level

- Loss of appetite

- Dry mouth

- Sleep issues

- Mixed senses (for example, "seeing" sounds or "hearing" hues)

- Spiritual encounters

- Feelings of unwinding or separation from self/condition

- Uncoordinated developments

- Lowered hindrance

- Excessive sweating

- Panic

- Paranoia - extraordinary and nonsensical doubt of others

- Psychosis - disarranged intuition disengaged from the real world

Bigger psilocybin dosages, including an overdose, can prompt extreme hallucinogenic impacts over a more drawn out timeframe. An extreme "trip" scene may happen, which may include alarm, suspicion, psychosis, terrible representations ("awful excursion"), and infrequently passing. The memory of an "awful excursion" can endure forever.

Maltreatment of psilocybin mushrooms could likewise prompt harmfulness or passing if a noxious mushroom is inaccurately thought to be an "enchantment" mushroom and ingested. In the case of regurgitating, looseness of the bowels or stomach cramps start a few hours subsequent to devouring the mushrooms, the chance of harming with poisonous mushrooms ought to be thought of, and crisis clinical consideration ought to be looked for right away.

Resilience to the utilization of psilocybin has been accounted for, which implies an individual needs an expanding bigger portion to get the equivalent hallucinogenic impact. "Flashbacks," like those happen in certain individuals subsequent to utilizing LSD, have likewise been accounted for with mushrooms. It is accounted for that individual who uses LSD or mescaline can construct a cross- resilience to psilocybin, also.

To What Extent Do Mushrooms Stay in Your System?

Regular psychedelic drugs, with the conceivable special case of phencyclidine (PCP), are not generally tried for on standard work environment medicate screens. In any case, whenever wanted by legitimate specialists, clinical workforce, or a business, it is conceivable to perform lab measures that can distinguish any medication or metabolite, including psilocybin, through cutting edge procedures.

At the point when tried through pee, the psilocybin mushroom metabolite psilocin can remain in your framework for as long as three days. In any case, metabolic rate, age, weight, age, ailments, tranquilize resistance, different medications or drugs utilized, and pee pH of every individual may influence real location periods.

Degree of Hallucinogenic Mushroom Use

In light of a 2018 review from SAMHSA's National Survey on Drug Use and Health (NSDUH), about 5.6 million individuals matured 12 or more established announced utilizing stimulants (which may incorporate psilocybin mushrooms) in the year preceding the overview. In 2017, that number was generally 5.1 million. In the review, stimulants incorporate psilocybin from mushrooms, yet additionally, other psychedelic medications like LSD, MDMA (Ecstasy, Molly), and peyote (mescaline). In correlation, 43.5 million individuals utilized cannabis in the year preceding the 2018 study.

In 2018, there were 1.1 million individuals age 12 and more who had utilized stimulants just because inside the previous year. Specifically, undergrads, and individuals ages 18 to 25, may pick mushrooms as a medication of misuse.

What Are Hallucinogens?

The concept was initially coined because they produce hallucinations but do not usually trigger them, at least at usual dosages. This name is, therefore, a misnomer.

Over the years, many different names were proposed for this drug class. In this century, the famous German toxicologist Louis Lewin used the term phantastica, and as we shall see later, the concept is far from too far-fetched. The best-known names – hallucinogen, psychotomimetic, and psychedelic ('mind-manifesting'). Nowadays, however, the stimulant is the most commonly used designation in scientific literature, although it describes the actual effects of such drugs inaccurately. The psychedelic concept is still the most common in the lay press and has continued for almost four decades.

Recently, there has been a trend in unsuspecting circles that acknowledges the potential of such drugs to bring forward supernatural experiences and generate feelings of spiritual meaning. Therefore Ruck et al. coined the term entheogen derived from the Greek word "ethnos," meaning "god inside," and it has been used more and more. This term indicates that such substances expose or require connections to "divine within." While it seems unlikely that this word would ever be recognized in formal science circles, its usage in the mass media and on internet sites has drastically increased. In fact, the entheogen has substituted psychedelic for the name of the choice in many of the countercultures which use these substances, and we should expect that trend to continue.

Chapter 3

Health Benefits Psilocybin Mushroom

Psychedelic mushrooms have a long-standing, deep, and tested reputation as a cure and change agent among the many historical cultures that they have used. Beyond all else, today, the advantages of these powerful little fungi are widely recognized. Studies are being carried out throughout the United States and abroad on the widespread and multifarious use of psychoactive mushrooms, and evidence is strong that they genuinely drive personal development. In addition, a recent study in the psychopharmacology journal found "there are major and lasting decreases in depressed mood and anxiety and improvements in quality of life with one single dose of psilocybin."

In addition, in traditional medical research, the mysterious and profound encounters experienced when psilocybin reached the American psychedelic lexicon in the 1960s have been studied and discussed. The results are promising and convincing and suggest that psilocybin can be a strong healer.

Clinical trials in the United States and abroad have been and are being conducted for patients dealing with life-threatening cancer. These studies primarily aim to clarify the efficacy of high-dose psilocybin interactions in recovery settings as a method to relieve psychological stress and anxiety, frequently following a life-threatening diagnosis. The results were promising so far. Under double-blind, placebo-controlled conditions, a single high dose of

psilocybin found that people with terminal diagnoses had fewer signs of psychological distress and important and lasting results.

In addition, a growing amount of research indicates that part of the impact of psilocybin is that it stimulates neuroplasticity or the capacity of the brain to learn, to develop, and, most significantly, to improve.

RISKS/HAZARDS

Psilocybin is considered largely one of the safest psychoactive substances. The 2017 Global-Drug-Survey found psilocybin the safest of all recreational products on the market, with a need for emergency medical therapy of just 0,2% of those taking psilocybin in 2016. This is five times less than MDMA, LSD, and cocaine. Psilocybin is also not addictive, and there is no known lethal dose, which means you are not likely to overdose although you are on a bad trip.

That said, taking any medication is not risk-free. Psilocybin can lead to certain physical side effects at the start and during a trip, such as nausea, suddenness, numbness, and tremors. It can also lead to fear, panic, paranoia, and changes in mood.

A journal published in Substance Abuse and Misuse found that sometime during their trip, up to 33 percent of the people surveyed who had taken mushrooms experienced paranoia and anxiety. Long-term effects are rare, both physical and psychological. Research suggests that the cause is latent psychological disorders rather than the mushrooms.

Nonetheless, there is something called Hallucinogen Persistent Perception Disorder (HPPD), commonly called "flashbacks." Moreover, HPPD is special to psychedelics and includes visual

changes within weeks or months of using psilocybin (or other psychedelic) as opposed to flashbacks associated with PTSD. The prevalence of HPPD is unclear, but it is considered to be a rare condition and does not require any physical or neurological changes.

MEDICAL USE

In the 60s and 70s, psilocybin studies have shown that psilocybin can play a significant part in the management and treatment of many disorders, including cluster headaches, mood, and addiction.

However, research on its therapeutic effects became virtually non- existent after the federal government had reclassified psilocybin into a Schedule I medicine in the 1970s. With the third wave of psychedelics, all this has changed.

With stories of the medical and regulatory effects of psilocybin, which finally capture the attention of medical professionals and regulators and lead into the mainstream, many firms, including The Johns Hopkins Center for Psychedelic & Consciousness Research, The Beckley Foundation, and MAPS, are now financing and conducting research. Work in the '60s and '70s has shown that psilocybin can have significant therapeutic effects.

-         Psilocybin Mushrooms Could Free the Mind Of Depression

A typical misinterpretation is that this mushroom enhances your present state of mind, so in the event that you are discouraged, in principle, it would aggravate it. This isn't the situation as indicated by introductory research 1, which found that enchantment mushrooms can improve the state of mind on a drawn-out premise.

It is important that these tests are directed in controlled and helpful settings. Gloom is a convoluted ailment; we don't prescribe attempting to repeat their discoveries outside of a clinical/restorative condition until more is known.

-    Psilocybin Mushrooms Can Help You Quit Smoking

As indicated by an investigation, psilocybin-based treatment can assist smokers with kicking their nicotine dependence on the control, with discoveries recommending it has an 80% achievement rate after only three meetings. What's more, we are talking completely dependent individuals here, who have been smoking a pack of day for quite a long time. To place it into the setting, one of the most achievement pharmaceutical other options, varenicline, just has a 35% achievement rate. The suggestions here are gigantic for the measure of life that could be spared.

It isn't only the situation of flying back a couple of mushrooms and being relieved – they are being utilized as a component of organized treatment.

- Psilocybin Mushrooms Prevent Cluster Headaches

Cluster headaches are one of the most difficult ailments known to man. It is depicted as having an ice-pack push through your skull and out your eye. For victims, it is a horrific experience, as it is a reoccurring condition that is exceptionally impervious to current medication. It is terrible to the point that it is frequently alluded to as "self-destruction migraines" the same number of have been headed to end their own life by the agony. All things considered, certain researchers presently accept that the appropriate response could be there in no time flat before us: psilocybin mushrooms. As indicated by narrative reports and starting logical perceptions, the utilization of enchantment mushrooms to treat bunch cerebral pains is very viable, placing numerous cases into abatement, and in any event, ending the condition for quite a long time at once.

- Psilocybin Mushrooms Contribute to Long Term Psychological Health

Recent research has demonstrated that the psilocybin in enchantment mushrooms makes the mind revamp itself, making new associations between neurons. This change isn't irregular or turbulent, however. Another request is delivered, making the sentiment of extended awareness. It makes it exceptionally simple to think "fresh" and permits us to see things from a totally alternate point of view.

The consequence of this is in spite of the fact that the excursion just keeps going a couple of hours, the disclosures and standpoints we gain remain with us for quite a while. The outcome is dependable constructive outcomes on our psychological prosperity. An extraordinary case of this is to inquire about from John Hopkins University. Not exclusively did most of the members in this examination express that the mushroom trip was one of the most significant encounters of their lives; they likewise announced an expanded feeling of prosperity 2 years after the fact on – something loved ones of members saw and concurred with.

- Psilocybin Mushrooms Help People Come to Terms with Terminal Illness

Realizing that you have a specific short measure of time to live is a very upsetting encounter. Psychedelics like enchantment mushrooms can enable terminal patients to manage their circumstances, diminishing uneasiness and ingraining a feeling of

harmony. It fairly follows on from the last point – permitting patients to see things from an elective viewpoint and leave them with a feeling of otherworldliness and prosperity. It can have the effect between spiraling into misery or investing your residual energy on earth, getting a charge out of the affection for loved ones.

Obviously, science has possibly truly started to expose what's underneath with regards to the possibilities of enchantment mushrooms. As research extends and clinical preliminaries become a chance, a wide range of new and intriguing applications could be found.

- Psilocybin in Mood and Anxiety Disorders Treatment

Psilocybin (and other psychedelics) have been shown for years to be an effective treatment for mood disorders such as depression and fear. Apparently, in the third wave of psychedelics, this is one of the most prevalent clinical areas of modern psilocybin research, allowing the federal government to conduct some small, highly controlled studies of the therapeutic potential of psilocybin in mood disorders.

For example, in 2011, a pilot study tested the effects of psilocybin in terminal patients with cancer on depression and end-of-life anxiety. Patients in this study had advanced cancer and a clinical diagnosis of their disease-related stress or anxiety. Studies have seen significant improvements in tests of depression and anxiety up to six months after psilocybin therapy. This research was eventually granted Phase II status by the FDA, which would allow for a larger study.

Another report from a leading London research group shows that psilocybin could be used to treat major depression.]

In the study, 12 patients were treated with two doses of psilocybin (one low and one high), along with psychological support. One week after the second dose, depression rates in almost all patients were significantly decreased, 8 of 12 showing no depression symptoms. Three months later, five patients remained depression-free, and four of the other seven were reduced from 'Severe' to 'Mild or Moderate' in their level of depression.

In small studies of people who did not respond to conventional serotonin reuptake inhibitor (SRI) drug therapy, psilocybin treatment has also successfully reduced symptoms of obsessive-compulsive disorders (OCD). In this study, all patients reported a decrease of 23% to 100% in OCD symptoms.

- Psilocybin in Addiction Treatment

In the '50s and '60s, "current psychedelics" were used to treat addiction with promising results in preclinical trials. Once again, however, work into their use for therapeutic applications stopped as many of these psychedelics were found illegal in the USA and most of Europe. Nevertheless, in recent years work has resurged into psilocybin and other psychedelics as potential therapies for dependency.

In a 2015 study, for example, psilocybin has been shown to be effective as part of a supported treatment plan to treat alcoholism. Significant reductions in beverage and drinking abstinence have been reported as part of a treatment program after psilocybin administration.

Psilocybin also appears to be a possible method for people to avoid smoking. In a recent trial, 15 smokers had two to three psilocybin therapies as part of a larger cognitive-behavioral reduction program. Twelve (80 percent) of the participants were successfully able to leave. In contrast, the success rates of the traditional quit method — including gum, patches, and cold turkey — are around 35 percent.

- Psilocybin in Cluster Headaches Treatment

Cluster headaches are often described as the most painful and disturbing type of headache but are shorter in duration than migraines and significantly interfere with a person.

There has been no systematic research documenting the effectiveness of psilocybin for treating cluster headaches so far, but anecdotal reports suggesting that this use has attracted the attention of the medical community. In the mid-2000s, psilocybin and LSD as possible treatments were identified by medical professionals after a certain number of their patients reported remission of their condition following therapeutic and psychedelic use.

One recent survey has found that psilocybin could be more effective than currently available medications when psilocybin is reported as a completely effective treatment. Many clinical studies are underway on this use, and further work should be available soon.

Does the Psilocybin Rewire Brain?

Many researchers continue to theorize that many of the beneficial effects of psilocybin on mental health disorders are due to the capacity of the brain control system to "reset" the Default Mode Network (DMN). An overactive DMN was associated with depression and other mood disorders, and psilocybin showed a drastic reduction in activity in the region. This was due to the effects of antidepressants.

PERSONAL GROWTH

However, the nicest aspect of the deliberate and conscientious use of psilocybin is its ability to promote personal growth. Many participants reported lasting beneficial changes in their personality behavior, values, and attitudes in early trials where psychedelics were given to healthy adults under supportive conditions. More recent studies also reflected these early results. Around 40 % of participants in laboratory studies involving psilocybin reported positive, long-term esthetic changes and changes in their relation to nature.

Such initial observations have since been followed by anecdotal accounts. In many cases, people report a greater appreciation of music, art, and nature along with greater tolerance of others and increased creativity and imagination, following a psilocybin experience.

More than one year after participants had a single experiment with psilocybin, their self-reported accessibility measure remained substantially high, researching a mysterious but strong dimension of the mushroom trip in this trial and beyond that.

A mystical experiment is characterized in this case as "the feelings of unity and interconnection with every person and thing, a sense of sacredness, a feeling of peace and happiness, a sense of transcendence of normal time and space, ineffectiveness and intuitive conviction that experience is an objective source of truth about the nature of life." In addition, research has shown that the more intense the mystical experience, the longer a person sees the positive and long-term changes.

Such subjective results, for example, feelings of interconnection, are possibly the product of the ability of psilocybin to decrease integration hubs in mind. In plain language, this means psilocybin allows for more "cross-talk" between typically segregated regions of the brain. Investigators speculate that this allows "uncontrolled cognition," which breaks down the ways we typically organize, categorize, and differentiate the aspects of awareness and flexibilities thinking. To understand how this can be helpful, it helps to know that specific patterns of brain activity are often found in different meditation states. For more about this, see our blog post about combining psychedelics and meditation.

It may, therefore, not surprise you that research has demonstrated that psilocybine can be used to improve one's spiritual practice. Seventy-five participants have taken a six-month spiritual training involving meditation, awareness, and self-reflection in a recent study. During the course, a low or high dose of psilocybin was administered to the participants. At the end of six months, the participants showed a substantial change in spirituality measures such as interpersonal closeness, the importance of life, death transcendence, and redemption, despite the high psilocybin dose.

In this regard, many people assume that psilocybin (and other psychedelics) can be an important component of self-improvement and self-optimization.

With the experience of feeling linked to the world (in some specific form) and meeting the deepest part of yourself, many believe psilocybin will help you take the measures you need to become the best version of yourself.

MICRODOSING

This is the act of consuming psychedelic substances sub-perceptually (unnoticeable). Many people with psilocybin mushrooms integrated into their weekly routine report more creativity, more energy, more focus, and better relationships, as well as reduced fear, stress, and even depression. Some enthusiasts also say that psilocybin micro-dosing helps them improve their spiritual consciousness and senses.

The modern-history of psychedelics stretches back to the 1950s; the publication of Dr. James Fadiman's 2011 book, Psychedelic explorer's guide: Safe, Therapeutic, and Sacred Journeys has given rise to the interest in micro-dosing. The book discusses micro-dosing as a psychedelic subculture. Whereas several indigenous and modern professionals have used microdosing to reveal a number of benefits, Fadiman's book has formally included the term "micro- dosing" in the psychedelic mainstream.

Fadiman's ongoing research is also one of the few modern studies specifically on the effects of microdosing. Although some recent clinical studies have examined the efficacy of microdosing, we know more about how large doses of psychedelics do for the brain. But it is possible that microdosing works similarly, only at a smaller level. Read our complete microsing guide to learn more about microdosing.

LEGALITIES

Psilocybin has been illegal for decades in most countries, but in some areas, it falls within a legally grey area. For example, in the Netherlands, you can buy magic truffles containing psilocybin without

breaking the law because of legal loopholes. Psilocybin is also legal in some form in Brazil, Jamaica, and the UK Virgin Islands.

While psilocybin is illegal on the federal level in the U.S., in 2005, psilocybin mushrooms were considered legal for cultivation and possession (unless dried) in New Mexico. In 1978, the Supreme Court of Florida decided that it was effectively legal to harvest wild psilocybin mushrooms before state lawmakers stated otherwise. Several new laws have been passed so far in order to control the cultivation of wild psilocybin mushrooms.

Citizens in Denver, Colorado, voted on 7 May 2019 to decriminalize psilocybin mushroom. This means for adults 21 and older that it is no longer a punishable offense to have them for personal use. But that doesn't make them legal. However, you could as well face criminal charges if you are found selling or sharing psilocybin champignons and probably even developing them. For the rest of Colorado, the legislation remains unchanged, at least for now.

Oakland, California, followed up with a change of its own in June of the same year: the Council members unanimously voted not just to decriminalize psilocybin mushrooms, but also all "theological plants," including indoleamines, tryptamines, and phenethylamines. As in Denver, this applies only to adults 21 years of age and older and does not include synthetic plant or fungal substances, such as LSD. However, unlike in Denver, the production and sale of particular psychedelics-including psilocybin mushrooms-are also decriminalized (or rather prioritized by law enforcement). Oakland is actually implementing a 'Grow, Gather, Gift' legalization framework, which encourages people to cultivate, collect their own, and donate their own plant medicines rather than establish a profit market.

In the United States, with the exception of three states, psilocybin mushroom spores are perfectly legal because psilocybin or psilocin do not contain the chemicals specifically regulated under federal law. Although the spores are legal, growing mushrooms from the spores are still considered illegal.

Chapter 4

Psilocybin Mushroom Dosing

Many factors contribute to the experience of psilocybin, including dose, mentality, and the personal chemistry of your body. With this in mind, every single journey is unique for the person, time, and place, and apparently no way to predict exactly what is going to happen. But you must plan for your journey by understanding the typical experiences and effects of psilocybin.

Psilocybin champagne is usually eaten in its entirety dried, and most people agree that they do not taste great. To mask the taste, some people brew the champagne into a drink, put it in Nutella or peanut butter, mix it in juice or smoothie, or smooth it, and drop it in capsules. Each of these ways has a somewhat different effect. For example, drinking mushroom tea will cause effects more quickly than eating them; swallowing capsules can have effected a little later.

Typical trips with a moderate dose of psilocybin mushrooms (1-2,5 g) are increased emotional experiences, increased introspection, and altered psychological function in terms of the transient state between wakefulness and sleep. Brain imaging studies also indicate a psilocybin trip is neurologically close to dreaming, which gives you a clear understanding of what you think when you have a psychedelic experience.

Literally, you can expect to experience perceptual changes, synesthesia, emotional changes, and a perturbed sense of time in a psilocybin experience. Perceptual changes, such as the halos in light

and objects, as well as geometric patterns when your eyes are closed, can include visuals. You can also experience vivid colors, tracers, distorted vision, and a feeling of the world around you.

Thoughts and feelings can also shift. It is not uncommon to have a sense of openness to thoughts and sentiments, as well as a sense of wonder and enjoyment about the world around you, the people in your lives, and your own mind. You might also experience a sense of peace and relationship with the world.

Strong, fun, and challenging emotions are normal during a journey. When unwelcome feelings occur, it is best not to fight but to encourage them to pass. Many people who report that strong negative emotions also feel calm acceptance and detachment at the same time, especially if they do not resist and remember that the emotions are temporary. Emotion resistance can lead to a "bad journey" (see "Bad trips" for more detail).

The effects of physical adverse events may vary from person to person but can include changes in heart rate (up or down), blood pressure changes (up or down), nausea, increased tendon reflexes, tremors, dilated pupils, restlessness or excitement and movement problems. Others say that they are deeply relaxed and calm.

A study also found psilocybin can lead to headaches lasting for healthy people for up to one day. However, neither of the subjects reported severe headaches, and psilocybin is actually used to treat a clinical condition called cluster headaches.

Psilocybin Effects

For psychedelic mushrooms, psilocybin is the active psychedelic component. The threshold dose for the sensation of the effects of

dried champignons is usually 0.2-0.5 g, but for each individual person, it varies. Usually, a moderate dosage from 1-2.5 g orally produces effects lasting three to six hours. Psilocybin is approximately 100 times less powerful than LSD and ten times less than mescaline.

When you take psilocybin, the body converts the drug into psilocin, which all contribute to psychedelic effects. Psilocybin and psilocin primarily interact with brain serotonin receptors and have an especially high affinity for 5-HT (serotonin) receptors of the 2A subtype. In rodents, psilocybin has shown strong interaction with sensory receptors in hub areas of the brain. This can explain effects like synesthesia — the experience of mixing sensory modalities, like hearing colors or sampling sounds — and changes sensory experiences on pillow trips.

Effect by Dose

Please take note that the effects listed below are not intended for the lower dose range in particular. They can be modified as more reliable, widely representative information is available.

The dosage ranges are for mushrooms of Psilocybe cubensis. They may apply to other species of psilocybin, but some species (e.g., P. semilanceata) on average are more potent.

- Microdose (0.05-0.25 g)

Microdose is a (not recognizable) sub-perceptual dose that many people take into their weekly routines. The concept behind this is that innovation, energy, and focus should be increased, and stress levels, anxiety, and emotional instability should be decreased. Find out more in our guide to micro-dosing. Common effects include the following:

• Mood improvement

• Reduced stress

• Control of the emotion

• Peace, mindfulness, and presence

• Openness and self-pity

• Fluidity of speech

• Alleviation of Impaired conditions like depression, anxiety, ADD

/ ADHD, and PTSD

- Increased motivation (e.g., positive improvements to lifestyles)
- Increased flow conditions
- Clearer, more related thinking
- Enhanced memory
- Enhanced creativity
- Promoting meditation
- Improved physical endurance
- Increased overall strength (without fear or crash)
- A slight increase in mood, positive or negative
- A possible state of sanity
- Increased neuroticism potentially

- Mini-dose (0.25-0.75 g)

Although an adequate microdose should not be felt, a mini dose of psilocybin takes you above the perception threshold — but not a complete journey. Simply put by one of the community members, a small dose gives you "the total increase of your being, the total sense of free flow" without losing contact with your surroundings. Common effects include the following:

- Mood improvement, slight euphoria or arousal.

- Peace, mindfulness, and presence

- Openness and self-pity

- Introspective opinions

- Alleviation of Impaired conditions like depression, anxiety, ADD

/ ADHD and PTSD

• Improved motivation (e.g., constructive improvements to lifestyles)

- Improved flow conditions

- Clearer, more related thinking

- Improved senses

- Promoting meditation

- Increased physical activity and daily tasks

- Preference for socialization introspection

- Increased light sensitivity

- Very soft visuals

- A possible state of manic

- Difficulty focusing

- Problems with other cognitive functions

- Fear, restlessness, or agitation

- Socializing difficulties or discomforts

- Museum dose (0.5-1.5 g)

The psilocybin effects are more apparent with a museum dose than with a small dosage, but the psychedelic experience in a museum dose is still not complete. The word "museum dosage," coined by Dr.

Alexander Shulgin, a biochemist, and pharmacist, points out that on this dose, you still can engage without any focus in public activities (like seeing paintings in the museum). Common effects include the following:

- Mood change, euphoria or arousal.

- Mild to moderate (e.g., "breathing" environments) visuals

- Enhanced empathy

- Fluidity of speech

- Introspection

- Improved flow conditions

- Enhanced senses

- Enhanced understanding of music, art, etc.

- Enhanced creativity

- Mood enhancement, positive or negative

- Altered sound perception

- Dilatation or contraction of time (time going slower or faster)

- Improved light sensitivity

- Dilation of the pupil

- Focusing difficulties or thinking loops

- Socializing difficulties or discomforts

- Dosage frustration ("no man's land")

-       Moderate dose (2-3.5 g)

This is the beginning of the full psychedelic experience. You will probably see visual hallucinations, with patterns and fractals, and things like the perception of time and depth will be distorted. Even with this dosage, you can still understand your surroundings – they

will only be significantly altered.
Common effects include the following:

- Introspective or philosophical insights to change life

- Increased ideas flow

- Increased understanding of music, fashion, etc.

- Consider funny or interesting stuff considered boring

- Clear up, top, and down

- Amplifying emotions, good or bad

- Visuals of the open and closed eyes (e.g. shapes, auras)

- Synesthesia

- Light sensitivity

- Compulsive yawing

- Distortion

- Fear and anxiety ("bad trip")

- Difficulty with cognitive functions

- Dizziness

- Nausea

- Megadose (5+ g)

A megadose leads to a total loss of links to reality. Intense visions, ego destruction, spiritual encounters and extreme introspection will be felt there. Common effects include the following:

- Magical insight and deep, wonderful feelings

- Introspective or philosophical insights to change life

- Death of the ego

- Really powerful visions of open and closed eyes (e.g. life coming memories)

- Synesthesia

- Time without purpose

- Distortion

- Impaired motor functions

- Strong fears and anxieties (extreme experiences of "bad trip")

- Extreme cognitive problems

- Dizziness

- Nausea

Additional Drug Interactions

There are not much data available about the relationship between psilocybin and other drugs, whether good or bad, but it is best to be careful and cautious when combining two substances together. This is what we know.

This is what we know.

Strong/Positive-Interactions

• Cannabis: This has the potential to enhance the mushroom's psychedelic character. But wait until the latter half of the experiment so that psilocybin does not interfere with the insight.

• Ketamine: The classic combination of Burning Man is Psilocybin + Ketamine. When you combine ketamine with psilocybin, wait until the duration of the sensation of psilocybin is over before you use ketamine.

• MDMA: Combining MDMA and psilocybin, known as "hippy flipping," is a common practice. While no current research supports the protection or danger of this combination, anecdotal reports suggest that MDMA may improve psilocybin journey and even lead to your avoidance of negative emotions.

Neutral-Interactions

• Coffee: There are no known side effects for coffee and psilocybin combination, but others claim the boost in strength of caffeine will enhance the perception of psilocybin.

Negative-Interactions

• Alcohol: Anecdotal reports from emergency areas say that the easiest and best bet is to abstain from alcohol while in mushrooms. Indeed, alcohol should be avoided while using any psychedelic.

•Adderall, Xanax, SSRI: These are powerful psychoactive drugs with largely subjective side effects and should be treated with extreme caution if you take any of these medications on a regular basis. Psilocybin is a potent serotonin agonist that can interact with other medications that alter the serotonin function.

CHAPTER 5

FINDING PSILOCYBIN MUSHROOM?

Psilocybin mushrooms are a favorite all-time psychonaut. We belong to a class of psychedelics known as entheogens – this term has been designed to describe their profound mystical properties and functions and can be translated as "demonstrative godhood."

There is evidence that Aztecs, Mayas, and other ancient Mesoamerican cultures have been used ritually in psychedelic mushroom and maybe even thousands of years ago by native Saharan tribes in North Africa. According to Terence McKenna, psilocybin might potentially grow our imagination hundreds of thousands of years ago.

In any event, people have connected with the divine through magical mushrooms for a long time and the tradition has evolved into the modern age. Within this modern era, however, the cultivation and use of shrooms in most parts of the world is forbidden by law. The problem arises, how and where will magical mushrooms be found? Without further detail, below are some of the most open ways to source it.

Choose Them Yourself

It might not be as difficult to find psychedelic mushrooms as you would think. The first place to look for them is perhaps the most obvious – your own backyard.

Mushrooms containing psilocybin are plentiful in nature. If you live in the right place, during their fruiting season, you can be very

fortunate. Nonetheless, you need to know the different strains that grow in your area seriously. It is understood that mushrooms are found in all shapes and sizes and at varying toxic levels. Others can cause moderate toxicity, whereas others may be very lethal. Often the variations in appearance are minute, but make sure you don't end up with what you're selecting.

Moisture is the number one element that all fungi need to grow. Dry air and wind can kill them easily. We do require a specific temperature, a fertile soil full of nutrients such as sugar, starch, lignin, fats, protein, and nitrogen, for growing species. If the tree bark, fallen leaves, dung, mucous, or compost have the right amount of nutrients, mushrooms will happily sprout on the surface. We don't need a dark atmosphere necessarily, but the lack of light allows the air to retain its humidity. This is why heavily forested areas surrounding large bodies of water usually provide suitable conditions, and it's an ideal place to look for them.

Animal dung (particularly cow dung) is as nutritious as it is – if the moisture is right, it is highly likely that it will grow out of it.

Psychedelic mushrooms can be found very widely in North America, especially the west coast, the north-east, and the Gulf of Mexico. We are packed with Mexico itself and much of Central America. Many countries like Ecuador, Colombia, Brazil, Venezuela, and Argentina also are so. Hawaii does not only appear to be a vacation paradise- other world-class strains come from these ancient islands. South Africa, the eastern coast of Australia, South India, the Philippines, and almost all of the coastal region of Southeast Asia are rich shrooms. Oh, and you can also find shrooms that expand throughout Europe.

Yeah, if you feel like you're smoking, the chances are that somewhere nearby, there are new magic shrooms. But again, make sure you get very familiar with, impact and appearance of all types of mushrooms in your field. Erowid has a helpful tool to classify the trippy, and Shroomery has a comprehensive list of all psilocybin shroom species found in countries worldwide and in the USA. Mycotopia is also an outstanding online forum where you can explore everything you are interested in or concerned about.

What to Look for When Searching for Magic Mushrooms

There is an enormous number of varieties of mushrooms in general, and the same is true for those that contain psilocybin. There are currently approximately 227 approved and listed species, 53 of which are cultivated in Mexico, 19 in Australia, 22 in the USA and Canada, 16 in Europe, and 15 in Asia. In terms of where they are grown, some of these species overlap, others are native to other areas and conditions.

There is no single feature that can differentiate magical mushrooms from normal mushrooms. They come in many shapes, sizes, and colors, and the only way they can really differentiate is by understanding their presence well and having the experience of champagne hunting.

A successful approach is to familiarize yourself with the most growing psychedelic shrooms in the wild. Here are the top five to continue with:

1.   Psilocybe subcubensis and Psilocybe cubensis are two species found all over the world in tropical areas. The former is much more common, being the most popular species of

magical mushrooms, while the latter is not so abundant but can be found in the same areas. They also have a very similar appearance: they are traditional, stubby, parasol-shaped mushrooms with mainly light-to-gold-brown caps, bulbous, wide and large in diameter, when fully grown, prior to the growth. A certain type of P. cubensis is worldwide known as the "Golden Teacher."

2.   Psilocybe semilanceata may be the psychedelic shrooms most widely available. In case you live in Europe, North and South America, Asia, Australia, and New Zealand, you will probably be able to find them. They are sometimes called 'Liberty Caps' because of their dark bell-shaped tops. Their stalks are slender and wavy.

3.   Due to its undulating tops, Psilocybe cyanescens are very easily identified. That is why they are usually called "Wavy Tops." These are among the strongest magic mushrooms in North America and hit a minimum of 1.96 percent of active compound content by dry weight. They often occupy a sufficient range of latitudes and are present in Central and Western Europe, New Zealand and parts of western Asia on the West coast of the U.S., in the South of the Bay Area.

4.   The "Hawaiian" shrooms of the Panaeolus or Copelandia cyanescens are not the most distinct species with long, slender stitches and small, brown to medium grey caps. Nevertheless, they are there with the greats in terms of their influence. They grow in all parts of the world: South America, North-South America, Western Europe, Central Africa, South and Southeast Asia, and all of Oceania.

5. Psilocybe azurescens is endemic to the western coast, Oregon, and Washington in particular. You win a spot in the top five because you will find almost the highest concentration of psilocybin among all magic champagne species: up to 1.80 percent. They also have an unbelievable amount of baeocystin which is a chemical psilocybin analog. Compared with P. cubensis, they can contain this compound by dry weight up to ten times more, which makes them one of the most powerful magic mushrooms. These are also pretty shrooms with a slender stem and a caramel-colored convex cap with a conical tip.

Growing Magical Mushrooms

If you are not seduced by the possibility of collecting research that could lead to misidentification-induced poisoning or you live in areas where magical mushrooms are not safe, you will be glad to know that there is a viable alternative: to grow shrooms on your own is fairly easy! Even better than that: growing mushrooms provide a year-round supply, enables you to try strains from around the world, and – best of all – if you are living in the US (not in CA, GA or ID), spores are legal for buying because psilocybin or psilocin is not yet present, as they are active psychedelic elements. If you live in NM, even mushroom growing is legal! See our detailed guide on the legality of mushrooms worldwide for more information.

There are two ways to do it – either you can order an uninoculated package and spores online, or you can make your own substrate on- line. The first option is easier – if your material comes from a reputable seller and no contamination occurs, all you will need is to keep your grow kit in a dark, wet place. However, we advise you to use DIY in this project – it's more fun, you can learn more from it, and it can produce better results. Fortunately, The Third Wave has established an easy-to-follow, detailed guide on how to do this.

Buy them in Countries that are Legal

A third choice is to review our guide to the International Legality of Psilocybin and to find nearby places where you can purchase, procure and ingest psilocybin safely and lawfully.

You have several choices when you're in Europe: the Netherlands, Austria, the Czech Republic, Spain and Portugal. In 2008, psilocybin mushrooms were naturally banned by the Netherlands, but magical truffles are perfectly safe to buy and eat. If you're interested in this, please check out our guide to the variations between natural and fake truffles. Psilocybin has undergone depenalization for the majority of the world, which means that it is only permissible to have limited quantities for personal use.

If you are searching for a more organized setting to legally and guardedly seek psilocybin, then you can find a directed psilocybin retreat in Amsterdam with our trustworthy partner, Synthesis.

It's everything there is to it. This book should contain sufficient information to start your mushroom-sourcing business. Make sure that you follow the law and remain secure in your quest and psycho- nautical activity, as always.

Chapter 6

Psilocybin Truffles And Psilocybin Mushrooms

Psilocybin truffle and mushrooms contain the same active compounds (psilocybin, psilocybin, and baeocystin), but vary in how they come from a very similar type of psychedelic. Psilocybin truffles are underground clusters that form from mycelial strands, while psilocybin champignons develop fully under favorable conditions.

However, they are made of the same material, they have some variations. Some of these variations are the most commonly asked questions:

• Are the truffles legal rather than the mushrooms?

• Are bubbles better than truffles?

• Are the travels qualitatively different?

• Are truffles safer than mushrooms?

Some of the most common and well-studied psychedelics are psilocybin mushrooms (aka Magic Mushrooms or Shrooms), with work in the early 1960s. Prehistoric people are believed to have been used for ritual purposes and to be responsible for the emergence of consciousness itself.

Psilocybin truffles are a more modern species that hit the mainstream market after the big 2008 repression of the Dutch government against psilocybin mushrooms.

To date, truffles are happily available in specialized shops in Amsterdam, somehow remained legal. The town was a stoner paradise forever, but the

Truffles declared a great tourist value for exploration of the conscience, as a psychedelic very available … or just tripping out.

If you live in Europe, Truffles can also be purchased online from our approved suppliers, web sites like Truffle Magic.

Psilocybin mushrooms and psilocybin truffles similarly affect consciousness. Symptoms often include perceptual changes, particularly visual changes, feelings of unity, or unity with everyone, a thorough understanding of the nature of life, and ego-dissolution.

Let us look at the basic facts of each one before we get to the differences.

BASIC FACTS

Psilocybin Mushrooms:

•   Used since 1000 BC by traditional societies

•   The average dosage is 10-40 mg, equivalent to approximately 1-4 g dried champagne.

•   Dozens of various types

•   The journey takes four to eight hours.

- No physical dependence potential

Psilocybin Truffles:

- Reputation gained following 2008 Dutch outlawing of champagne

- They were on the market before that but made no sales

- Produced in order to avoid mycelial growth through control conditions such as temperature and moisture

- Sold typically in 15 g boxes labeled with strength

- The journey is from 3 to 5 hours.

- No physical dependence potential

Are you interested in not psychoactive mushrooms' health benefits? Four Sigmatic looks for additional mushrooms and beverages.

PSILOCYBIN 's General Effects

- Runs into self-drop and a sense of self-esteem and world harmony.

- Encourages the feelings of a positive bond between nature and the world.

•   It can send the impression that emotions can be unpredictable on the fence between a positive journey and a bad one.

•   Typically going up is crazy. Usually, come down relaxed and content.

•   The sober reality can be lost during a journey. Perception and orientation can dramatically change and make it difficult to understand where you are and what is happening.

•   May cause a feeling of melting and unable to move around. It is also recommended that during the trips, you should sit on a comfortable surface.

•   Triggers incredible visions in the closed eyes. Fascinating open-eye hallucinations and auditive echoes are also possible.

•   There may be an over-stimulation of senses, and further stimulation is seen as an unnecessary intrusion. The best environment is a secure and quiet place without loud music and potential intruders.

•   Offers the potential for a deep, introspective journey and new insights into life and prospects.

Differences Between Mushrooms and Truffles

Although the psilocybin and psilocybin mushrooms both contain the same active ingredients, there are several differences in their content:

Legal

Since the psychedelic substances contain the same active ingredients, the rest of the world recognizes mushrooms and truffles as illegal narcotics. However, Holland is one of the very few countries in Europe to have psilocybin in limited quantities, lawfully or decriminally, and it is the only country that makes a distinction. With both illegal psychonauts in the rest of the world, they usually choose mushrooms, which are more prevalent and considered as an immersive voyage.

Trip Intensity

The main difference between them and the Dutch government's most likely cause for not banning them is their size. Although scientific precision is hard to tell, especially given that there are so many different types of truffle and champagne, anecdotal reports on trips to the Truffle usually describe milder events with less pronounced hallucinations and a more preserved activity and sociability functioning. The senses are not overcharged. In the stimulating environment of downtown Amsterdam, users do not seem to have problems consuming truffles.

It must be stated here, however, that both are identical chemically. There is no clear explanation of why a high enough dosage of the truffle doesn't cause the same intensity as the mushrooms even though the concentration of the active compounds is different.

This may also be that the use of truffles is more standardized – when it comes to packets of a fixed size, with a clearly labeled intensity and an explanatory guide (to be followed by the friendly dealer's normal advice words), truffles are less likely to be overviewed.

Nature of the Trip

Trips to truffle are generally called "fun," while experience in champagne is often described as "deep and introspective trips." While qualitative differences in the nature of experience are not theoretically acceptable, the lighter the effect of truffles seems to be more carefree.

While there are degrees of distortion of perception, the universe does not seem to be that different. The enlarged field of view is there, but it may not be all around and it may be funnier than amazing truffles in comparison with mushrooms. Similarly, while the horizontal or perpendicular position is probably the most convenient, you may have no problem walking around the lake to marvel at the suddenly magical pebbles and trees they sound like alive.

Chapter 7

Lysergic Acid Diethlyamide (Lsd) And Psilocybin Mushrooms

The most commonly used psychedelics are probably LSD and psilocybin mushrooms (also called "shrooms" – psilocybin is the main ingredient). However, many people wonder about the disparity.

The following common issues are:

•   How do the LCD and psilocybin mushrooms feel? Do psilocybin mushrooms feel 'natural' rather than LSD?

•   Are visuals different?

•   Are psilocybin mushrooms more stable (or vice versa) than LSDs?

•   How to consume LSD versus psilocybin mushrooms?

•   Any difference between LSD and acid?

However, the mainstream use of LSD was popular in the 1960s, psilocybin champions have been used for centuries in the shamanic traditions.

Psilocybin mushrooms and LSD have commonalities, like all psychedelics, as they influence human consciousness. Visuals, feelings of isolation or alienation and self-elimination are typical symptoms.

However, there are significant differences as anybody who has used both LSD and psilocybine champignons will tell you.

Quick Facts On Lsd And Psilocybin Mushrooms

•   Micrograms psychoactive (millionths a gram)

•   LSD is the short name for Lysergic Acid Diethlyamide chemical compound

•   LSD is also known as 'acid' and sometimes tabs are known as doses which describe blotter tabs to which the LSD is used.

•   In 1943, it was first used and it was synthesized in 1938

•   A fungus that grows on rye is derived from ergot

•   Typical 100 to 250 micrograms dose

•   The trip last abour 8-12 hours.

•   No physical dependency potential

•   LSD is a component under Schedule I under the Controlled Substances Act declared illegal in 1968.

Psilocybin-Mushrooms

•   Used from 1000 BC

•   Psilocybin is usually supplied to 10-40 mg, which corresponds to approximately 1-4 g of dried champagne.

- Dozens of psilocybin-containing various mushroom types

- The journey takes 6 to 8 hours.

- No physical addiction potential

- Legally available to buy in form of truffles made from psilocybin

- Decriminalized anywhere in the United States

'The LSD vs psilocybin champagne what am I going to do? '

Every personal experience varies, however, anecdotal reports show overlapping phenomena.

You can prepare your own experience using these studies. Please note that this is because of moderate dose consumption (LSD: 100-

250 micrograms – 2-4 grams psilocybine mushrooms).

Approximately 1/10th of a moderate dose, microdosing with these materials can lead to different effects.

Lsd Versus Psilocybin Mushroom Effects

What are LSD 's Effects?

- Facts more practical. Easier, if possible, to connect with sober people. Also contributes to a "super" experience.

• Increased risk of being positive. Bubbling users, constructive energy fills users.

• Users record a less emotionally charged LSD experience than psilocybin champagne.

• Setting and setting extremely sensitive. You 're much more likely to have a successful trip by managing these two variables.

What are Psilocybin Mushroom Effects?

• Brings about ego-drop and absolute universe peace

• Many consumers feel closer to the natural world in mushrooms with psilocybin

• On the fence of good and bad trips, emotions are volatile and inconsistent.

• "Come up" can be quite intense

• Users report more introspection, losing touch with sober reality

How to Take Psilocybin Mushrooms and How to Take LSD?

The LSD is typically a liquid or a paper, gel, or breadcrumbs that has been filled with liquid LSD. Paper tabs are most commonly left to dissolve under the tongue. Psilocybin fungi are usually consumed in a dried form, or ground into powders and added to a food or drink in capsules.

The principal difference is the flavor. The flavor. Pure LSD should be unflavored, and psilocybin mushrooms have an unpleasant taste. All LSD and psilocybin champignons are vulnerable to Queasiness, which may also be attributed to empty stomach and frowning nerves.

LSD and Psilocybin Mushrooms: How Long to Get Started? And How Long Does It Last?

In addition to the longer-lasting LSD effect (up to 12 horas compared to 6-8 hours for champagne), both drugs have different start times and progressions. At the beginning it is not too clear, but the LSD is a bit faster than psilocybin mushrooms, which usually take about 1 hour. This is about 30-45 minutes.

You appear to "sing" with mushrooms around 80 minutes after ingestion, while an LSD may occur for several hours. An LSD journey is also long enough to produce many peaks, while psilocybin mushrooms usually last only for a significant peak.

Visual Effects: LSD and Psilocybin mushrooms

Psilocybin mushrooms are more likely to develop psilocybin in terms of visuals than LSD. The use of LSD is rare with hallucinations. With LSD, objects or surfaces are often viewed as throbbing or as "breathing" and traces of moving objects can be seen. The visual effects of LSD are similar to its cognitive effects, so objects appear clean and smooth while remaining real, and colors appear more vivid.

Psilocybin mushrooms have stronger visual effects, where static objects are shifting or changing, and whole objects are sometimes pictured. Color may be heavily influenced and all colors that merge

into a cohesive theme or pattern — a purple or sepia lens, for example, can appear to make the entire world look.

Mental and Physical Effects of LSD and Psilocybin Mushrooms

The LSD and psilocybin champagne mental effects are also quite distinct. LSD definitely changes and alters perception, but it somehow maintains even in depths of uncertainty a paradoxical sense of consciousness.

It is much more likely to feel unregulated and disconnected from your sense of yourself and daily thought with psilocybin mushrooms. This can be cool but also disturbing and intense.

LSD appears to induce restricted and anxious energy in a physical sense. Sometimes you have to move around physically to help control it, or it becomes anxiety or restlessness. The physical effects of Psilocybin mushrooms are more rooted. You are strong, strongly rooted and, in particular, deeply connected to nature when outside. These drugs also have beneficial effects on the relation between mind and body.

Several site quotes that explain the difference between LSD and psilocybin mushrooms creatively are discussed here:

• "You feel like driving your car in cocaine, you feel like you are on the backseat for the ride with psilocybin champagne."

• "Acid feels like you're plugged into the universe while shrooms are like a forest old tree."

• "Champs are used to set up your roots. LSD is used to spread branches."

• "The psilocybin mushrooms, in my opinion, are more likely to cause mental drawbacks.

In many respects, they are an entirely different ballpark. Mushrooms do not have clarity, LSD's 'perfection,' yet they do have a specific quality that often leads to a deeper inspection.

• "LSD is simplified ... It makes me more mentally aware, with greater exposure and insight into my own feelings ... Shrooms are fine seed ... It makes me feel nice, powerful and overall. They're taking you with them.

• "This is a quite big difference because LSD does not have much body travel or at least not a comparable ... LSD is far more brain." • (On the "high body" of psilocybin mushrooms).

• "Shrooms have a much more drug-friendly feeling for me. With a little bit of tripleness, I always get a rush like MDMA.

What About Both?

LSD and psilocybin mushrooms may definitely be mixed. But that can be challenging. The two drugs are always too strong and the individual loses comprehension and control. It is important that all substances are dosed correctly.

It is highly recommended to first get acquainted with each drug separately if you suggest trying LSD and mushrooms together. A good beginning would be to reduce the dosage of each single substance by approximately one third and be prepared for an intense experience.

The trials of LSD and psilocybin mushrooms are a host of success stories, which reinforce the sharp and clearness of LSD in its unique visual effects and loopy mood. But it is worth a separate test if the two substances are successfully mixed. There is still a big question:

Which of the Psychedelic Should You Try?

Many say that LSD is at first easier to manage. This also leads to an atmosphere that is more optimistic, and many find that consistency and focus are more friendly.

On the other hand, psilocybin mushrooms can be preferable for those who seek an intense, grounded, and visually stimulating experience. It's more "earthy" and rooted and can take you away from your "self" in many respects. It may be daunting and not necessarily bad.

It is always best to turn your first encounter into a meaningful one because of the variable and daunting nature of psychedelics.

You should be prepared, research and enter if you want to try LSD or psilocybin mushrooms for the first time.

Chapter 8

Preparing For Psychedelic Trip?

In this chapter, we want to make sure that you have a good ride on your first rabbit hole. Religiously follow these important guidelines, whether you just want to giggle uncontrollably for a while or give wings to your spirits.

Your first mushroom or truffle trip is supposed to leave you with the "wow" factor. It can and should be a life-changing, spiritually enhancing, and a great adventure of self-exploration. Getting it right from the beginning will ensure an enlightening, euphoric, and wonderful experience.

The first shroom trip could be a great, a great and life-changing trip. However, it can as well be vicious, taking control of your world and your senses, throwing you into a terrific, horrible psilocybin mushroom world, a bad-trip.

As a popular dietician would say, "set and setting" has a lot to do with the one you end up with. Yet, there are lots of other factors that influence the shroom trips, including the dosage, the species of magic mushrooms, and simply the wills of your subconscious brain. Anyone new to magic mushrooms should learn before they trip (if you're someone I'm talking about, good job; you're reading this!), but as they grow more experienced, they're going to learn how to take psilocybin mushrooms in the right way, to make a good, if not a wonderful, snorkel trip.

Magic Mushrooms Chemical Structure

Well, if you've heard (or even heard) about the effects of acid or LSD, the psilocybin-shroom trip is basically the same, with a different "edge" to it. Part of the known background to this fact is that both psilocin and psilocybin, as we know that these two are the psychedelic compounds in shrooms, as well as acid, are either confirmed as partial or full agonists at different serotonin receptors (the agonist is a chemical that activates the receptor in the body, and practically the antagonist is basically the one that makes a reversal of its effects) throughout the brain.

Psilocin and psilocybin have similar chemical structures to the A.K.A. 5-HT serotonin chemical, although the 3D shape of the LSD is quite different.

What Are Magic Mushroom Trips Really Like?

There is a myth floating around that magic mushrooms, as well as LSD, do not cause "hallucinations;" they simply "distort" what you see using your senses. Apparently, this is what shrooms and acid do today at average doses. However, at much higher, aka "spiritual," doses, intense hallucinations, as well as magic mushroom trips and acid trips, will envelop the world around the tripper as they lose themselves to the world of psychedelics.

With lower doses, the shroom trip on some Sativa is much like impossibly high. Firstly, the colors of objects become vivid and saturated, making them "clear." Euphoria will take over, and then nothing will happen, giggling and smiling over absolutely nothing. Sounds are likely to repeat again and again, and then you may not be sure if the sound actually happened in the first place.

When you're able to feed, the flavors are vivid and foreign, and you can also change the flavors of your mouth when you chew.

Yet this is the first part of it. Closing your eyes now, you will see intense geometric patterns, 3-dimensional, sliding, rotating, and morphing through various complicated structures. Open your eyes widely, and on the sides of the walls, on the floors and ceilings, on the rocks, and on the furniture, you will see the patterns in their full light that continue to change in their complexity.

Then come the thoughts. Many characterize it as a feeling of "independence," as if the barrier that separates the conscious and subconscious was unexpectedly shut down. Loads of thought will gush freely and easily, without effort, taking their own paths, sometimes even splitting up into two completely separate sequences of thought, occurring simultaneously until they re-emerge again.

Close your eyes now, and if the dosage is right, absolute, life-like hallucinations will take over your mind's eyes, consume your senses, and carry out all the stories that your subconscious takes to the table.

Somewhat at this stage, which can be reached by someone with no magic mushroom tolerance of only a minute to average dose, some shroom trippers already have a "clear understanding on their roles in life" as well as, in some cases, conversations with divine beings or intelligence beings of "different dimensions" or worlds.

How Can I Have A Great Magic Mushroom Trip?

First and foremost, every person responds differently to various medications, like psilocybin mushrooms. And this why it so imperative to start small, feel the world of mushrooms, and judge for yourself how much you're going to take next time.

With that in mind, decide how serious your first series of trips are. Will, you ultimately want to dive into your subconscious brain, float through the various environments while integrating different definitions of life; or do you just want a sweet, soothing magic mushroom high with some fun, tactile, and fascinating shapes? You're going to need to stock up accordingly, based on how many trips you're going to have and how much you want to take, but hang on, we're going to get a dosage of psilocybin mushroom in just a second.

Getting Set

Before you even begin to think about the intensity of the trip, the dosage, and think about it like that, you need to establish a safe, calm tripping environment, i.e. Timothy Leary's "up and go." For most of you, that doesn't involve going out on the streets or in the woods or washes, but in a house where you can experience the journey, walking outdoors if you want to enjoy the beauty of nature.

Getting set also requires a state of mind. Then, do not start consuming psilocybin mushroom the day before you get an exam or an interview. Also, do not pick a safe house where someone you don't want to know about using your shroom is likely to show up (or is already there). A mixture of anxiety and annoyance before a trip can quickly turn into a frightening, chaotic, bad trip. Always be calm, enjoy the shroom experience with an open mind, and know that whatever comes in, you'll be all right. And you're going to be.

Get a Trip-Sitter

The trip sitter is the way to make sure that you're actually going to be all right. Find a trip site or a sober person who has the time and experience to take care of you, to help you with your magic mushroom experience. Most often than not, most trippers who take psilocybin mushrooms more than once end up figuring that experiencing a trip sitter helped them out, whether it was just giving them a blanket when they wanted one or whether they ended up protecting the tripper from police trouble or worse, physical damage. So if you trip on psilocybin shrooms, take a trip.

What If the Trip Is Not Going Well?

Perhaps it's your first time going on a psychedelic trip, or maybe you consider the end results of your mushrooms to be a little too intense. No need to worry!

The Trip Stopper 3000 helps mitigate the consequences of a poor ride for a quick comedown. In case you have Trip Stopper 3000 within reach, it will make you more comfortable so you can better enjoy your mushroom trip!

1.   Take two white capsules (maltodextrin) to alleviate the effects of your journey.

2.   Take two dark capsules (valerian) to relax.

3.   Eat something savory.

4.   Keep calm, breathe slowly, and realize that the bad feeling will soon pass.

How Many Magic Mushrooms Should You Take?

If you have the set and set up worked out, you have a nice time with a buffer explicitly set aside for the shroom ride, and you've got a good trip-sitter on your side, it's time to start considering doses.

After this, doses are good guides, according to Erowid, for new to medium magic mushroom users. More novice shroom trippers will have built up a reasonable tolerance and would therefore want to adapt accordingly; however, being a novice shroom tripper, luckily, you know how to judge your own body well enough. Interestingly, the doses are practically dependent on the Psilocybe cubensis.

Light-Dose

The Erowid Vault says about a quarter of a gram of dried magic mushroom is a threshold dose. A threshold dose is a dosage that will have a shroom user just barely feeling the impact. A trigger dose of psilocybin mushrooms often gives a faint sensation of cold along with a mild vividness of colors and faint, but not much more.

The dosage page goes on to state that a "light dose" of psilocybin mushrooms is about a quarter of a gram, the reference dose, to about one gram of dried shroom.

Some peoples' eyes will dilate at this stage. Sensitive trippers may feel a bit of the classic mushroom nausea kick in at this point.

Slight visual "hallucinations," but they are more like flickering illusions, can start to reveal themselves at the bright colors and the edges of peripheral vision, and vivid lights can take on a" starry " appearance, according to the website. The distinct "mushroom aura "is noticeable.

Low Dosage

A " medium "portion, Erowid notes, is around a gram to more than two. Be that as it may, note, everybody's mushroom experience will be unique. Numerous individuals feel no a larger number of side effects than they would from a little portion biting down over two grams of shroom just because, while others taking that sum have stumbled hard, hitting an all out psilocybin experience total with distinctive pipedreams and spinning musings. The best activity here, in the event that you 're not certain the amount you need to take, is to begin at around a gram and a half, or even a light portion in the event that you 're had a history being touchy to hallucinogenic.

At medium doses, physical impacts will be completely obvious, including the shroom queasiness for touchy trippers and apprentices. Understudies are plainly widened at this stage, and circulatory strain and pulse will increment to a sheltered degree.

Numerous clients state the " cooling "feeling experienced at edge dosages get more grounded as the excursion advances. Out and out, open peered toward visuals please now, and the fantasy like pictures of shroom outings will begin to come to fruition.

Numerous individuals concur that, with a medium dosage, their idea designs are definitely extraordinary; it 's workable for " illuminated " feelings and clear acknowledge about the universe to show. Simultaneously, feelings can be unpredictable and intensified, and outrageous emotional episodes among rapture and dysphoria that mirror the emotional episodes of LSD will happen.

Strong Dosage

At long last, the dosage page depicted " solid doses "as anyplace among more than two to five grams of dried mushroom, with more

than five grams of shroom recorded as a " substantial" portion. Magic mushroom learners that need to encounter a genuine, full mushroom trip regularly take-up to an eighth of an ounce (around three and a half grams) on their first portion, and the excursion can be an euphoric, educational encounter.

However, at trip forces moving toward that point, an awful outing can get, well, awful, and new shroom clients who aren't accustomed to adapting to terrible excursions can be in for an unpleasant time. In the event that a learner is moving toward this level of solidarity, they likely overdosed (this implies, just, to take more than expected; overdoses don't show that demise or other perpetual physical mischief is done), and the commencement of the shroom outing will be unexpected, difficult, and most likely not charming. Students would be little and substantial, and queasiness will unleash total destruction on a tripper 's stomach now; even prepared magic mushroom clients would make some hard memories in the event that they weren't set up for the size of the effect.

In correlation, if a psychonaut is hoping to accomplish the stage and is totally arranged for what it offers, enormous doses might be exceptionally euphoric and life changing in a significant manner. Psilocybin, in exceptional doses or taken in intense magic mushrooms, can likewise cause an encounter known as " inner self misfortune, " which is essentially the loss of the sentiment of one 's " self. " The " sensation "of self-image misfortune is regularly characterized as a negligible charge with one 's world, being lost in the flow of the outing with no focal want, strife, or influence. Frequently, it 's called being "one" with the world.

What Number Of Magic Mushrooms Can I Buy?

This is a sensitive issue. The appropriate response is none. You truly shouldn't accept mushrooms purchase the number, except if you're a psilocybin mushroom producer purchasing seeds (and in the event that you are, at that point, why understood this?). You should get them by the gram or by the ounce. Also, in the event that you 're genuine about not being ripped off, you'll either purchase from somebody who looks at the shrooms on a scale before you, or you'll approach one so you can test the entirety yourself. No, you ought to approach a scale at any rate, to weigh out doses, yet many individuals will pull off eyeballing the heap of shrooms on the off chance that they realize the amount they've requested.

In case you're intending to trip a couple of times, you don't have to get yourself in excess of an eighth of dried shrooms, and you could do with even less (as usual, this all relies upon the strength of the magic mushrooms your source load up on). This being your first ride, you likely won't gain admittance to individuals who purchase psilocybin mushrooms by the mass, and your contacts will be insignificant.

Be glad having an eighth for around $30 or €20 to €25 for your first shroom buy, or around $10 to $15 or €8 to €10 a gram, if that is your purchasing gadget. Individuals who trip in some cases commonly by psilocybin mushrooms by quarter ounces, half ounces, and ounces or more, getting paces of about $100 to $200 or €75 to €150 per ounce, and it's normal for some hallucinogenic lovers with solid associations with request or be without given doses.

In case you simply need to pass judgment on the measure of magic mushrooms you 're jumping on the spot, just by taking a gander at them, you can figure around ten to fifteen individual mushrooms to

weigh about an eighth of an ounce. In you have the opportunity previously, simply check Google for "an eighth of shrooms " or something like get a view on what it'll outwardly resemble. In general, be that as it may, it's additionally best to look at your doses, and in case you can get to a scale in any capacity, do it.

Chapter 9

Growing Psilocybin Mushrooms

This chapter is based on the eponymous PF Tek of Robert "Psylocybe Fanaticus" from McPherson — the method which revolutionized indoor mushrooms growing in the form of vermiculite (as opposed to grain alone), which gave the mycelium more space to grow and imitate natural conditions. Although his approach is a little more labor-intensive than others, it is also better suited for beginners because of its simplicity, low cost and reliability. It also utilizes products and ingredients that are readily available, many of which you already have.

- Spore Syringes

One thing you might find difficult is a good spore syringe. This will produce and "drop" the magic mushroom spores into the substratum. Some farmers have reported pollution problems, misidentified strains, and even water-free syringes. However, you should have no problems as long as you do your research and find a reputable supplier.

For all cases, after you have produced your first mushroom sample, you can start filling your own syringes.

What Kind of Variation Do I Choose?

You will want to settle on a species and strain as you learn how to grow champignons inside. The majority of providers offer a choice, but Psilocybe cubensis B+ and Golden Teacher mushrooms are one of the most popular for beginners. While not as strong as some

others, such as Penis Envy, the sub-optimal and changing conditions they apparently forgive are more.

What Will You Need?

Ingredients

• Syringe Spore, 10-12 cc.

• Flour of organic brown rice

• Medium / fine vermiculite.

• Drinking water

Equipment:

• Small nail and hammer

• 12 Shoulder-less half-pint jars (e.g. ball, jelly kerr or canning jars)

• Measuring cup

• Bowl for mixing

• Strainer

• Heavy duty foil (tin)

- Big tight cover pot for steaming
- Small towels (or about ten towels of paper)
- Tape micropore
- Transparent 50-115L plastic storage box
- ¼a-inch drill bit drill
- Perlite.
- Bottle of Mist Spray

Hygiene Supplies:

- Air sanitizer

- Rubbing alcohol
- Propane/butane torch lighter
- Disinfectant
- Latex gloves sterilized (optional)
- Surgical mask (optional)
- Glove box or still air (optional)

Instructions:

The basic PF Tek method is quite simple: prepare your substrate of brown rice, vermiculite and water and divide it among sterile glass jars. Enter spores and wait until the mycelium forms.

This is the filament network that supports your mushroom production. Move your colonized substrates or "cakes" to a chamber of fruit after 4-5 weeks and wait for your champagne to develop.

NOTE: Always ensure proper hygiene before beginning: spray the air sanitizer, disinfect your equipment and surfaces thoroughly, take a shower, brush your teeth, wear clean clothes etc. You don't need much space, but you should have as sterile an atmosphere as possible. In the conditions of cultivating shrooms, opportunistic bacteria and molds can proliferate so that the risk is minimized.

STEP 1: PREPARATION

1.   Prepare Jars:

• Knock four holes down around each of the cloves with the hammer and nail (which should be cleaned with alcohol to disinfect).

2.   Preparation of the substratum:

• Add ⅔ cup vermiculite and ¼ cup of water in the mixer for each glass. Use the disinfected strainer to remove excess water.

• Apply ¼ cup of brown rice flour to the bowl with a half-pint jar and stir with moist vermiculite.

3.   Fill Jars:

• Be careful not to stack too closely, fill the jars within half an inch of the rims.

• Sterilize the top half inch with alcohol rubbing

• Top off your bottles with a dry vermiculite layer for contaminant protection of the substratum.

4.   Sterilize steam:

• Screw the clothes securely and cover the tin foil of the bottles. Place the edges of the foil around the surface of the vessels so that the holes do not get water and condensation.

•   Put small sheets (or sheets) into the big pot and place the jars on top, so that they do not reach the floor.

•   Add tap water to a level the jars and boil slowly , making sure the jars are upright.

•   Place the tight lid on the pot for 75-90 minutes and leave to steam. If the pot is dry, fill it with hot tap water.

NOTE: Some farmers prefer a pressurizer set at 15 PSI for 60 minutes.

5.   Allow it to cool:

•   Leave the foil-covered jars in the pot several hours or overnight after steaming. Until the next step, you must be at room temperature.

STEP 2: INOCULATION

1.   Prepare and sanitize syringe:

•   Use a lighter to heat the needle length until it is red and hot. Allow it to cool down and dry with alcohol so that your hands do not touch it.

•   Squeeze the plunger and shake the syringe to disperse the magic mushroom spores uniformly.

NOTE: If your spore syringe and needle need to be placed before use, take great care to prevent contamination. The surest way is by placing the syringe in a disinfected quiet air or glove box, sterilized latex gloves and a surgical mask.

2.   Inject spores:

•   Remove the foil off the first of your jars and attach the syringe to one of the holes.

•   Inject around 1/4 cc of the spore solution (or slightly less if you use a 10 cc syringe on 12 jars) by touching the surface of the container.

•   Repeat the other 3 holes and clean the needle between them with alcohol.

•   Cover the microporous holes and hold the pot, leaving the foil off.

•   Repeat the process of inoculation for the remainder of the bottles, sterilizing with the lightest needle and alcohol.

STEP 3: COLONIZATION

1.   Wait for the mycelium:

•   Place clean and out of the way your inoculated jars somewhere. Remove direct sunlight and outside temperatures 70-80 ° F (room temperature).

•   White, fluffy-looking mycelium should start to spread from inoculation areas between seven and 14 days.

NOTE: Watch for signs of infection, including strange colors and smells, and immediately remove suspicious bottles. Do this outside in a dry bag without pulling out the cloths. If you are uncertain if a container is infected, always be careful — even if the substrate is otherwise colonized healthy — as some pollutants kill humans.

2.   Consolidate:

•   Have at least six successfully colonized jars after three to four weeks if all goes well. Let the mycelium hang on to the substrate for another seven days.

STEP 4: SETTING UP THE GROW CHAMBER

1.   Make a fruiting chamber shot gun:

•   Take your container and drill 1/2-inch holes, about two inches apart, on both sides, on the base and on the wall. To avoid cracking, drill a hole into a block of wood from the inside.

• Set the box to four stable objects arranged underneath at the corners to allow air to flow. You will also want to cover the surface underneath the box to protect against leakage of moisture.

NOTE: The fruiting chamber for a shotgun is far from the best design, but it is easy , fast and good for beginners. You might want to seek alternatives later.

2. Perlite added:

• Place your perlite under a strainer and run it to soak under the cold tap.

• Allow it to drain until no drips remain and scatter over the base of your chamber.

• Repeat for a perlite layer approximately 4-5 inches deep.

STEP 5: FRUITING

1. "Birth" of colonized mediums (or "cakes"):

Open your jars and remove from each layer of dry vermiculite, so as to avoid damaging your substrates, or "cakes."

Insert every jar and tap the disinfected surface to release the cakes.

2.   Ensure to Dunk the Cakes:

•   Rinse the cakes under a chilly tap one at a time to remove loose vermiculite, again to avoid injury.

•   Fill your cooking pot with tepid water or any other large container and put the cakes inside. Submerge them with another pot or similar heavy object just under the water.

•   Allow the cakes to rehydrate at room temperature for up to 24 hours.

3.   Roll the Cakes:

•   Remove cakes and put them on a disinfected surface from the water.

•   Fill the dry vermiculite of your mixing bowl.

•   One by one prepare the cakes to be coated with vermiculite. This helps to maintain moisture.

4.   Move to the grow chamber:

•   For each of your cakes, cut a square of tin foil, large enough to rest without touching the perlite.

•   Spread these uniformly in the growing chamber.

•   Place the cakes on top and mix the spray bottle in the chamber gently.

•   Before closing fan with the lid

5.   Optimizing and tracking conditions:

•   Mist the chamber about four times per day so as to keep moisture up, be careful not to water your cakes.

•   To increase airflow, fan with the lid up to six times a day, particularly after misting.

NOTE: Some farmers are using 12-hour fluorescent lighting, but indirect or ambient lighting is perfect during the day. Mycelium requires just a little light to see where the open air is and where mushrooms are to be made.

STEP 6: HARVESTING

1.   Watch out for the Fruits:

•   The mushroom or fruit appears as tiny white bumps until they sprout into "sticks." They 're ready to harvest after 5-12 days.

2.   Choose your fruit:

•   Slice the mushrooms close to the cake to remove when ready. Don't wait until they finish their development, as they start to lose power as they mature.

NOTE: Mushrooms are best picked just before the veil falls. They will have small, conical caps and covered gills at this stage.

STORAGE

Psilocybin mushrooms tend to go bad in the refrigerator within a couple of weeks. So, if you're going to use them for microdosing or just want to save them later, consider storage. Drying is the most efficient form of long-term storage. This should keep them strong for two to three years, while keeping them cool, dark, dry. If stored in the freezer, they will last almost for a longer time.

One of the best ways to dry your mushrooms is by leaving them outside on a sheet of paper for days, perhaps in front of a fan. The problem with this approach is they're not going to get "hot cracker." In other words, you're not going to break when you try to bend them, because they still hold some moisture. They can also raise their power dramatically, depending on how long you leave them out.

The most successful approach is by far the use of a dehydrator, but it can be expensive. A good alternative is to use the following desiccant:

•   Air your mushrooms dry 48 hours, with a fan preferably.

•   Growing a desiccant coating in the airtight container frame. Silk gel kitty litter and anhydrous calcium chloride are readily available as well and can be purchased from hardware-stores.

•   Ensure to put a wire rack or similar set-up over the desiccant so that you don't touch the mushrooms.

- Arrange your fungi on the rack, make sure that they aren't too close and seal the container.

- Wait a few days and then test to see if the cracker is dry.

- Switch to storage bags and put in the freezer, e.g. vacuum sealed, ZipLoc

RE-USING THE SUBSTRATE

After the first flush, the same cakes can be re-used up to three times. Just dry for a few days and repeat step 5.2 (dunking). But don't roll them in the vermiculite; only bring them back into the growing chamber and as before mist and fan. In case you begin to notice contaminants (usually around the third re-use), make sure you spray the cakes with a spray and dispose it outside in a secure bag.

HOW TO MAKE SPORE SYRINGES

It is just as auto-sufficient to fill your own psilocybin spore syringes.

Second, you have to take a spore print from a mature mushroom, i.e. one that can expand until its head opens and the edges up. You will also note a build-up of dark lilac deposits around the surface. These are the magic mushroom spores.

Remove the cap with a flame-sterilized scalpel to collect them and position it on a sterile sheet of paper. Cover with the disinfected glass or container and leave for 24 hours. to shield from the rain. Keep out of light in an airtight plastic bag the resulting spore print.

Scrape the spore print into a clean glass of distilled water to fill a spore syringe. This is available in auto parts shops. Also, fill your sterilize syringe (which should also be sterile) and regularly empty it into the glass to disperse the spores uniformly.

Fill it up for a final time and put it in an airtight plastic bag. Leave the spores to hydrate for a few days at room temperature. Then, you can as well keep the syringe in the refrigerator until you are ready to use it. It will last two months or more.

ALTERNATIVES AND ADAPTATIONS

Many changes were made to the PF Tek method to increase yield and to facilitate things. Often, with different substrates and environments, different species tend to perform better.

The principal alternative to the basic PF Tek is the monotube method of spawning coir, manure, straw or some other fresh, nutritive substrate into bulk. You may want to experiment with some of these other methods, but for now the PF Tek is a good introduction.

FREQUENTLY ASKED QUESTIONS ON HOW TO GROW PSILOCYBIN MUSHROOM

Question: How long does it take for magical mushrooms to grow at home?

Answer: The time it takes to grow growing fruit in a mycelium- colonized substratum depends on a variety of factors.

But the entire process of mushroom cultivation will take 1-2 months.

Question: How are we going to harvest shrooms?

Answer: You will be able to harvest your fruits 5-12 days after the first mushroom substratum starts to sprout.

They are harvested until the veil splits, i.e. before the veil fully matures and releases the spores. In other words, the gills still have to be covered. However, your mushrooms should also have light conical caps at this point.

Question: Where can a spore syringe be produced?

Answer: There is an instruction on how to create a spore syringe above. A sterilized knife and/or scalpel, a sterile sheet of paper, a disinfected glass or jar are needed to collect spores of psilocybin

from a mushroom that matures. Add the champagne spores to a glass of distilled water and load your sterile syringe. After a few days to hydrate at room temperature, it can be stored for at least a few months in the fridge.

Question: How to cultivate spore-less mushrooms at home?

Answer: If you don't want to add the spores yourself, use a Psilocybe cubensis growing pack. The standard cubensis kit comes with an already colonized substratum for the cultivation of mushrooms. We are available for various cubensis and specific animals.

Yet enchanted mushroom kits are not without critics.

Question: What's wrong with a magical mushroom growing kit?

Answer: Despite their apparent convenience, magical mushroom kits are commonly regarded as money waste. While they work at about the same price as from scratch, their content and quality are unknown. These may also be more vulnerable to pollution.

They cannot even work through user comments. At best, the findings are contradictory. Apart from something else, you won't learn how to cultivate magic mushrooms from scratch with a cubensis.

Question: What is the best substratum for mushrooms?

Answer: Although the brawn rice flour and vermiculite substrate have been tried and tested by generations of mushroom farmers, it may not be the best choice for everyone. It's up to your expectations. Brown rice flour is ideal for bulk production, but coir can be cheaper and easier to use. There is also entire brown rice (not flour), which is supposed to produce more potent fruit.

Another good choice is pasteurized manure, which is high in phosphorus, nitrogen and potassium. Throwing coffee grounds into the mix (up to one quarter of the entire mix) may help accelerate colonization. Spent coffee grounds are economical too; 99% of the coffee biomass not in the cup is usually thrown away.

Some farmers claim that the best substratum for champagne is filled with nutritional diversity. But too many nutrients from too many sources can lead to pollution. As a novice, you better keep it simple

– not to mention cheap enough for trial and error.

Question: What is the difference between magic substrate and mushroom spawn?

Answer: When you know more about growing mushrooms indoors, the terms "spawn" and "substrate" would often tend to be used interchangeably or incorrectly.

Simply put, when used to colonize a second, "Bulk substrate," (coir, manure, etc.) in the fruiting chamber, the substratum (the brown rice flour/vermiculite cakes in the PF Tek method) will become 'spawn.'

When you fruit directly from the cakes, as this guide says, the mushroom substratum remains the substratum after extracting it from the bottles.

Question: What are the best strains of Psilocybe cubensis?

Answer: The B+ and Golden Teacher mushrooms are some of the most common P. cubensis strains (or varieties) for beginners. Experienced growers may prefer Penis Envy.

Nonetheless, the best cubensis strain for you depends on your preferences for growing mushrooms as with your choice of

 substrate.

Question: How to Grow Magic Truffles?

Forget about growing mushrooms in a box; truffles are mostly grown in jars in place of a chamber of fruit. The use of a boiled-rye grain (aka rye berries) substratum is also a major difference to the PF Tek as described above.

Pana and P. tampanensis, also known as 'philosopher's stones,' are common truffle varieties.

Question: Where can I find supplies for growing mushrooms?

Answer: However, one of the great things about the PF Tek system is the large availability of supplies. You can find what you didn't already lie in the house in your local hardware store.

Your first load of psilocybin spores is the one thing you need a professional manufacturer. Forums are the easiest way to locate a credible one.

Chapter 10

How To Prepare Psilocybin Mushrooms For Microdosing

WHY MICRODOSING WITH PSILOCYBIN MUSHROOMS?

In case you are of sustainable orientation and don't have easy access to an organic chemicals laboratory to synthesize-LSD, microdosing with psilocybin mushrooms is a natural choice. While it's an easy way to microdose with LSD to snip or dilute blotter tabs, it means reliance on an external source that may be standardized or unreliable. You'll be in charge of the process by buying legal psilocybin truffles or even better by growing your own psilocybin mushrooms, and if you have a golden-brown thumb, you can take care of your mushroom microdose friends too.

Psilocybin mushroom microdosing is ideal for a psychonaut who loves to take part in every step of the process. Psilocybin for microdosing requires a little investment in kitchen equipment, but for around $80 you can easily buy anything you need.

If you have fresh psilocybin mushrooms, especially if they are cute miniature pinheads that never matured (see picture), you might be tempted to consider the "microshrooms for the microdosing" line.

There's something inherently organic that makes you feel that your coffee and your cereal just need to take a mushroom cap in the morning.

It will, however, most likely lead to inconsistent microdosing of psilocybin. Taking into account the following:

Fresh and dry psilocybin mushrooms, the 10% dry to wet ratio, are generally considered equivalent. Know, however, this is a reminder and fresh champagne can be more or less than 10% of their dry weight. That means that you can take more than 0,3 dry grams from 3 grams of fresh mushroom, depending on the mushroom and environmental factors, like humidity levels.

Caps and stalks contain different psilocybin levels. Psilocybin content in Psilocybe cubensis, one of the most commonly used strains, in the whole mushroom is 0,37–1,30 percent and in the head, 0,44–1,35 percent and in the stalk is 0,05–1,27 percent. In other words, the caps are on average slightly stronger than the stems and there are small bits of the stems with almost no psilocybin. In order to equalize, you will still ground your champagne to a fine powder.

The contents of psilocybin vary from champagne to mushroom, from flush to flush and between strains.

Changing varieties during your microdose regimen will make calibration difficult, because with each type of psilocybin mushroom you must consume a variety of psychoactive substances.

The content of psilocybin changes in the different stages of mushroom development. Miniature pine heads that have not grew larger can be stronger per gram of weight than large mushrooms.

However, you should be aware that dried truffles often contain less psilocybin than dry mushrooms when microdose – see weighing and measuring for different quantities you need to use.

Under-microdosing yourself is much less a concern than over- microdosing unintentionally. When you try to sort out the laundry list, finding yourself in touch with the stucco on the ceiling is not only unproductive but can raise your anxiety.

STORING MAGICAL MUSHROOM AND TRUFFLES

Successfully growing magic truffles and mushrooms are only a halfway, so you have to store them properly if you want to keep their power!

There are a few items more exhilarating and thrilling than picking the first flush of magic mushrooms or truffles.

Seeing the product of your efforts ends up creating a satisfying feeling and offering you a much more personal relationship to the material that will carry you through your trip. You 're not yet out of the jungle, though.

It can be a difficult business to store your magic mushrooms and truffles if you don't know how to do it correctly. It is very easy to damage them, reduce their contents or allow them to decompose. That is why it is a necessity for any aspiring psychonaut to learn how to safely and efficiently store them.

MUSHROOMS AND TRUFFLES STORAGE

Storing fresh mushrooms and truffles properly is relatively straight forward. Both can be kept loose up to a month in a quiet, cold location like your fridge. The temperature that will be needed is between 2-4 degrees Celsius. Mushrooms and truffles are also best placed on unbleached kitchen paper. A refrigerator is inherently moist, and excess humidity can lead to damage. Most of this danger is minimized by putting them on kitchen paper.

If a month isn't long enough, then a food vacuum packer may be purchased. Once vacuum is packaged and stored in a refrigerator, truffles last up to three months. In order to avoid bacterial growth, mushrooms must first be properly dried.

MAGIC DRYING AND TRUFFLES OF LONG-TERM STORAGE

In case a very long-term storage solution is needed, yet both magic truffles and mushrooms could be dried-out and safely stored in a cool and dry place for up to 2-3 years (maybe even longer). The only threats are insect infestation, and possible lack of potency due to exposure to light, moisture and fire. This works because mushrooms stop decomposing without their moisture content.

The trick of drying magical mushrooms and truffles is not to use heat. It is a common error, and sometimes used to try to speed up the operation. However, magic mushroom active compounds can be quite sensitive to long periods of heat, destruction and reduction of power.

The drying method for your magic crop includes pre-drying it to eliminate excess humidity and then a rigorous dry main using a desiccant. This will remove all available moisture and make your champagne and truffle ready for long-term storage.

In our helpful tutorial you can learn how to do this in even more depth. Even though it doesn't speak of truffles, it may use the same method.

MAGIC MUSHROOMS and TRUFFLES FREEZING

When you don't dry long enough, you might go an additional mile and freeze the mushrooms and truffles.

To do so, obey the advice above and test our guide to dry them absolutely. Before they are

frozen, both truffles and mushrooms must be fully dry. When cold, place it in a plastic zip bag and put it in your freezer. Frozen mushrooms and truffles may be kept pretty much forever.

IMPORTANT: Always freeze fresh magic truffles and mushrooms, this will destroy their cell membrane function, which has significantly diminished strength.

So, there you are! By now, you have known how to diligently store your magic truffles and mushrooms, also ensuring that their quality is maintained and that they are ready for use whenever you need them!

HOW TO STORE MAGIC MUSHROOMS

New mushrooms and truffles can be kept for up to a month comfortably in the refrigerator at 2-4 degrees Celsius. They should be bundled in a packet of paper or wrapped in a towel. The cool and dark environment of the refrigerator is good for conservation, but the moisture in the refrigerator will eventually affect the bacteria 's growth and decomposition. This applies in particular to mushrooms. Truffles will comfortably last for three months due to their lower moisture content, if the vacuum is sealed in a zip-lock container. Nevertheless, they must first be properly dried in order to preserve psilocybin mushrooms for longer.

Drying mushrooms eliminate moisture and any possibility of the formation of bacteria. This can be achieved in different ways. The methods range from putting them on the towel, putting them before a fan, to placing them in a box of Epsom's salts for several hours (this is a classical error, as any heat will decrease its power).

The complete and proper drying process involves a pre-drying phase, where the champions are placed under a dark tube or in front of a fan in the sun for a couple of hours before their texture becomes rubbery and their appearance wrinkles. A desiccant must then be added. This can be either a custom Epsom salt cooking or plain silica gel packages. The drying of the mushrooms is gradual; it takes a couple of weeks for the crackling state of complete dryness.

Nevertheless, for space, energy and time savings, a low-heat food dehydrate is one of the most efficient ways to preserve psilocybin champagne while retaining its strength. A dehydrate can set you back only about $40; and if you don't use it as a decoy that can make banana chips, it can double as cracker-dry portals. Various mushroom harvests can be dried in a de-hydrogenator overnight instead of being left over all surfaces of your home for weeks. For wet climates, dehydrators are particularly recommended.

When it has been fully dried, all mushrooms and truffles can be safely stored in a cool, quiet, dry place and for a couple of years, or even longer (if in this time frame one can not lose or consume them). The loss of power should be minimal to zero if the psilocybin inside is not lit, low or dry.

BEST WAYS TO PREPARE PSILOCYBIN MUSHROOMS FOR MICRODOSING

The best way of delivering the most consistent psilocybin microdose is by far to dust your dried psilocybin mushrooms. By melting together your mushrooms, you homogenize the variance in psilocybin contents between caps and stems and between mushrooms and mushrooms.

Fast note on the drying of mushrooms: The methods vary from towels to fans and low heat for several hours in a stove (this is a classical error, as heat will decrease their power), to Epsom salts.

The easiest way to make psilocybin champagne is by using a spice or coffee grinder. Unlike the dehydrator, a separate microdoser should be used, as all the small mushroom particles cannot be separated from the blades. Although it is fun to imagine your roommate enhancing her unintentionally when melting chai tea spices, it is best not to avoid unnecessary microdosing.

Practical tip: It takes less than a minute to pulsate into a fine powder in your psilocybin mushrooms. Do not open the grinder for a minimum of half an hour to let the fine dust settle in the chamber.

When this is opened right away, agitated particles will be sucked into the air in a whoosh of psychedelic fairy dust and ungather your kitchen for hours with the lasting smell of magic fungus. However, always remember that cannabis is not the only thing that gives you a buzz for ambient vapor inhalation.

WEIGHING AND MEASURING

An electronic scale is a fine starting point for the kitchen. Accurate measurements of 0.1 – 1.0 grams are roughly $20. Until pulverizing, weigh out dry mushrooms to see how much total mushroom mass is when powdered. Knowing how much you must first helps you to split the quantities for each microdose.

For example, after powdering 2 grams of dried whole mushrooms will produce 10 microdoses of 0.2 grams.

You need about one-tenth of a standard dose to microdose mushrooms. This means that you will use dried psilocybin

mushrooms at a dose between 0.2 – 0.5 grams. (Use between 0.5 –

1 gram of dried powdered truffles per dose if you are using psilocybin truffle – psilocybin would be less than psilocybin).

Always remember that this amount can be higher or lower depending on the neurophysiology, weight, and strength of each individual's mushrooms or truffles. A significant part of the microdosing process is to calculate the dose to match you exactly. This can take up to several microdoses, so it is best to begin low and then up (patiently) before you find your sweet spot with psilocybin.

In general, if you have a regular microdose of 0.2-0.5 g of mushrooms, you'll want to start with 0,1 g if you weigh less than 100 lbs. If you weigh about 200 lbs, however, you can start at 0.3 grams comfortably. Double these initial truffle doses. Here you can find a useful dosage calculator tool.

Sometimes, kitchen scales are not accurate to 0.1 grams. You can not register weight until it is at least 0.5 grams, which may be excessive for one microdose. Instead, simply add all of your powder to a piece of paper and micro-pile it evenly.

The problem with powdered mushrooms, as you will notice, is that its low density makes the powder float everywhere. So try not to breathe too much air as before, or you will have an aerial microdose.

In case that you do not want to divide your powder manually, there are other ways to distribute microdoses:

• Mushroom Capsules: For this, you will need a capsule filler dispenser. Such contraptions, which cost about 240 dollars, will charge several capsules simultaneously by distributing the powder equally around the capsule holder. This is a common

method for engaged micro (or macro) doses and has the benefit of overcoming the loamy mushroom taste not enjoyed by all. The disadvantage is that the quantity that fits into the capsules is predetermined and your tablets are ready to be measured. This makes it more difficult to adjust the dosage once you pack up your mushroom pills. Therefore you can use this form only if the perfect dose has been calculated. If you do, you can mix the mushroom powder with cocoa or powdered sugar in quantity required to fill the capsule and sustain the desired psilocybin microdose.

• Micro scoops: Just place all the powder of your mushroom in a small bowl and use a small spoon (1/16 - 1/8 of a teaspoon) to measure your doses. The benefit of this approach is that you can change the dosage on the go more flexibly and can do it even if there is no scale. The downside is that it is more susceptible to eyeballs.

• Combination: Use small scoops to measure and load into your capsules your psilocybin microdose. This is the way to flavorless microdose mushrooms with the flexibility to change the dose per need.

TAKING PSILOCYBIN MICRODOSE

Once your micro-dosage has been measured, there are many ways of ingesting it. We already have the option of a mushroom pill; Mushroom tea is the popular alternative, or you can decide to make a creative mix of your mushroom or truffle powder and, ultimately, whatever you eat every day.

Mushroom tea is very easy to make and reduces the flavor, especially if you add sweetness. Like any other tea, it is made. Only

pour hot water over the mushroom powder and blend until homogeneous. You can also add your microdose to your morning shake or blend it with the maple syrup you put on your pancake or add it to your brownies with chocolate icing. The chances are endless.

IMPORTANCE OF MICRODOSING FOR MUSHROOMS

Some take the powder only as it is. You may also apply it to your coffee or tea but the powder is water-insoluble and clumps into tiny pockets in your cup. Sprinkling cereal is a way to mask the earthy taste, mixed with orange juice or a spoonful of honey. Don't just throw it down the hole, whatever way you want! Be aware of your microdosing motives while using your dose. Microdosing provides the best results if you know why you are doing it

FREQUENTLY ASKED QUESTIONS ON MICRODOSING OF MUSHROOMS

Question: What Type of Magic Mushrooms can be Used for Microdosing?

Answer: You can use any type; most people choose classical strains Golden Teacher (Psilocybe cubensis) or Caps of Liberty (Psilocybe semilanceata). Since the small dose has a subperceptual effect, the strain should not be explicitly different. You took too much if you notice some effects; try dialing back the dosage until your sweet spot is found.

Questions: What's Best for Microdosing (Truffles or Magic Mushrooms)?

Answer: Both are approximately the same except the dose. Truffles have a lower psilocybin content, so a bigger dose is required.

Question: What are the Best Ways to Consume a MAGIC MUSHROOM?

Answer: Due to its precision, mushroom pills or capsules with an exact dose of mushroom powder are the best solutions. You may otherwise insert the powder into your tea, coffee, hot chocolate, smoothies, or other favorite drinks or eat it with sweetness, yogurt, cereal, or any other way.

Question: Can I Grind Magic Mushrooms without a Grinder?

Answer: And though no other method is as precise (and accuracy is important for microdosing), you should follow the old method and use scissors to pulverize them as finely as possible. A highly accurate digital scale would be critical in this situation because a second degree of imprecision would be applied to the dose fraction.

Question: What If I Consume Too Little or Too Much?

Answer: You won't notice anything if you take too little. When you take too much, you can experience somnolence or mental hyperactivity, depending on the pressure. The key is to find the dose just below the point where an effect occurs.

Question: Is Microdosing Mushrooms Safe?

Answer: It has been shown that taking appropriate (meaning not very high) doses of psilocybin is completely safe. Of course, taking a microdose is also safe. However, longitudinal research has not been done on regular microdosage for a long time, so we advise everyone not to microdose for more than a few months at a time.

Question: Can Mushroom Microdose Be Detected in a Drug Test?

Answer: Majority of standard drug tests do not include psilocybin and its metabolites. Often, however, they are included in extended screens

Chapter 11

Healthy And Tasty Magic Mushroom Recipes

In this chapter, we will discuss magic truffles - they are a gritty and soft, chewy, and even somewhat zesty. Be that as it may, we comprehend not every person is that partial to growth, so we thought of 5 delectable plans to dress them up:

Quite a number of mushroom lovers really appreciate yummy magic truffles - they are a natural and soft, chewy and even somewhat zesty. Be that as it may, we comprehend not every person is that attached to organism, so we concocted 5 scrumptious recipes to spice them up:

- Chocolate truffles

The old clans of Mexico and Central America were the primary individuals to find the intensity of the Theobroma cacao seeds. The Word is, even in those days, the Aztecs used to blend their magic mysteries in with what they called chocolate - an early form of today chocolate. In any case, chocolate is held in the most noteworthy respects - even the word theobroma truly converts into „food of the divine beings". However, this is a direct result of the invigorating impacts of theobromine - a compound firmly identified with caffeine - that chocolate and truffles go together so well.

For best outcomes, utilize great, crude and natural chocolate. Get the darkest chocolate you can discover. To liquefy the bar into a cream, utilize a twofold kettle or a griddle, yet be mindful so as not to

consume the chocolate. At the point when it's prepared, empty the hot cream into a shape - any sweets form or icecube plate will do - and allow it to chill off however much as could be expected without it getting hard. Blend in some finely slashed truffles and put it into the cooler to let it solidify out.

Truffles don't care for heat, so try to let the chocolate cream chill off enough before blending them in, else they could free their intensity.

- Truffle Tea

Truffle tea is an extraordinary method to expend the magic, as tea is more delicious and simpler to process than new or dried truffles. For some, tea is the favored technique to ingest them. First, to make the tea, slice the truffles in to exceptionally little pieces, or squash them up cautiously. That will help expand the surface territory so a greater amount of the dynamic substances will be discharged. Heat some water to the boiling point and let it chill off for 15 - 20 minutes. After, blend in the truffles and mix incidentally for around 5 minutes. Strain the tea and appreciate! To improve up, simply include somewhat nectar or sugar.

- Healthy balls

This conveys a good portion of protein and can be effectively arranged without heat. Besides, you can include your fixings and test with the taste as you want. As a fundamental formula, blend all in a significant bowl: moved oats, raisins, nutty spread, ground flax seeds, coconut drops, cocoa powder, nectar, cinnamon a little vanilla powder, and obviously - finely slashed magic truffles. Blend all fixings until they are equally appropriated, fold the balls, and put them into the cooler to solidify out—Presto - magic vitality balls.

- Yogurt squeezed orange and chai

This is basic. Simply blend your finely slashed truffles into an organic product yogurt (cherry works best to cover the parasites flavor!), in a glass of squeezed orange or some chai tea. The preferences mix well and you won't notice a very remarkable truffle taste when drinking.

- Capsules

In case you genuinely need to attempt magic truffles, however, can't get over the taste, at that point this is for you. Before you can make containers, you totally need to initially dry, and afterward, pound the truffles (best in an espresso processor). View our veggie-lover containers. They are made of pure vegetable cellulose and come in two sizes. Note that it will take more time for the truffles to produce results, since first the cellulose dividers need to break up in the stomach. To speed it up a little, simply take a needle and punch a couple of gaps into the case.

-       Be Creative!

Simply recollect that magic truffles don't care for heat - however, other than that, there's actually no limit to whatsoever you can do with them. Add them to a smoothie or milkshake? Shouldn't something be said about nectar drenched with almonds?

Chapter 12

The Most Famous Psychedelic Mushrooms

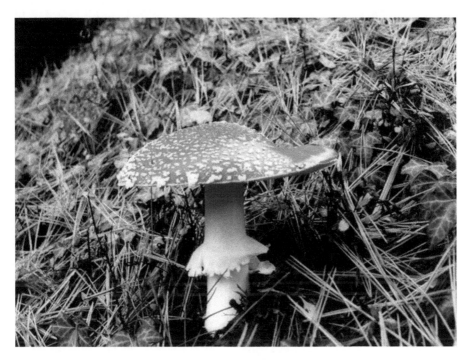

Amanita Muscaria (poisonous)

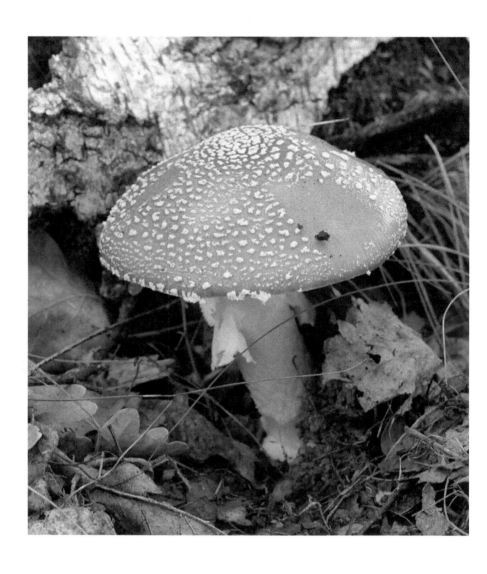

Amanita pantherine(poisonous)

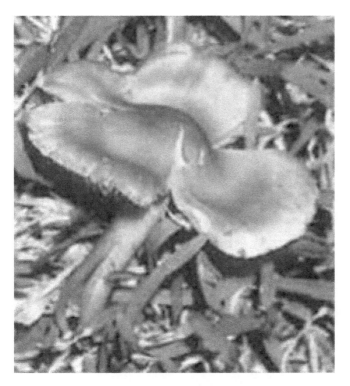

Inocybe aeruginascens(edible)

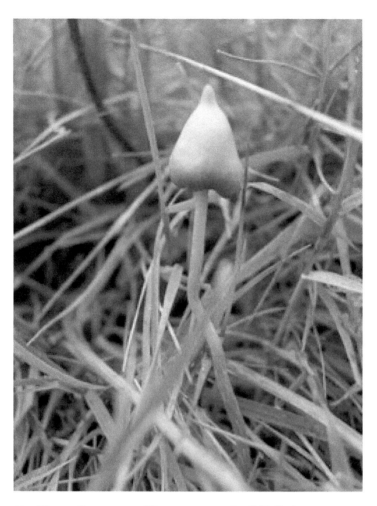

Psilocybe semilanceata(edible)

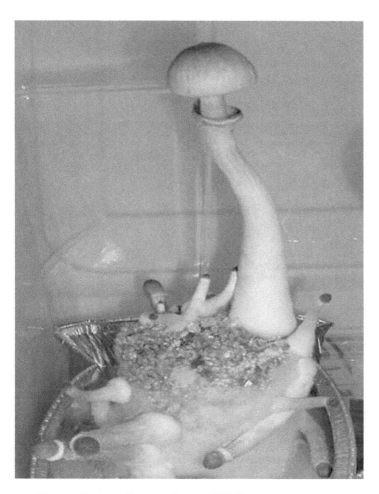

Psilocybe cubensis(edible)

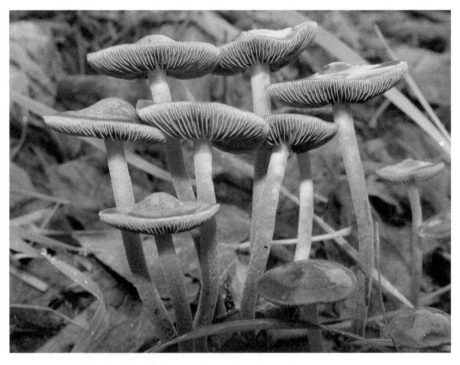

Panaeolus subbalteatus(not edibles)

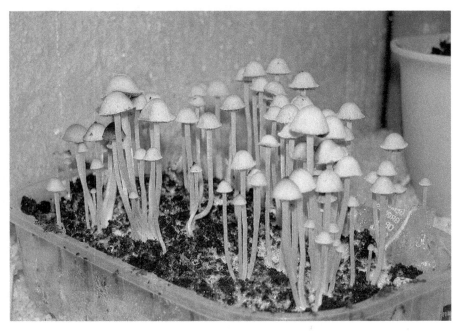

Panaeolus cyanescens(not edibles)

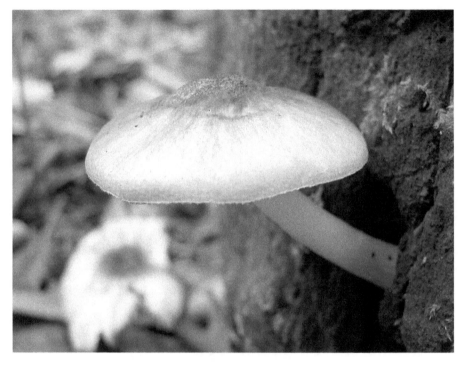

Pluteus salicinus (edibles only in you cook it)

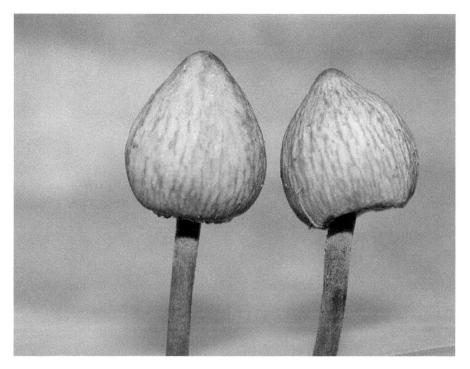

Panaeolus papilionaceus(edible)

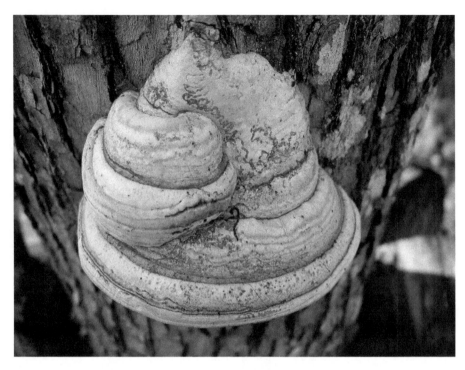

Fomes fomentarius(not edibles)

Conclusion

If you've made it to a point in this wonderful piece, you probably want more. We do learn about a limited number of people who have eaten and actually left Psilocybin cultivated to the wonders of the mushrooms.

Mushrooms of Psilocybin can allow you to dream, perceive, and see new things. In the next few days, please keep in mind any observations you might have had during your trip.

The mushrooms themselves will not change your life immediately, but you will find your life positively changed if you make the trip an enjoyable experience and don't dismiss the trip as just stupid fun.

The journey will become a catalyst for a host of positive changes. Keep your finger crossed and see.

Lightning Source UK Ltd.
Milton Keynes UK
UKHW021159280322
400721UK00009B/2225